THE

WRINKLY

RANCH

Unbelievably funny, shocking
and poignant anecdotes of life
and work in Long-Term Care

TRISTAN SQUIRE-SMITH, RN

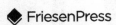 FriesenPress

One Printers Way
Altona, MB R0G 0B0
Canada

www.friesenpress.com

ISBN
978-1-03911-998-7 (Hardcover)
978-1-03911-997-0 (Paperback)
978-1-03911-999-4 (eBook)

1. MEDICAL, LONG-TERM CARE

Distributed to the trade by The Ingram Book Company

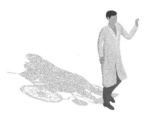

DEDICATION

To the majority who demonstrate grit and commitment to your colleagues, day in and day out, and who, no matter what, keep showing up—*thanks for coming in.* I am grateful for you being there for your peers and all who depend on the important but thankless work you do. I recognize and appreciate your unique and discretionary efforts.

... and to the others, the few who flake out and call in "sick" repeatedly—*go fuck yourselves.*[1] Do us all a favour and find another job; you're obviously not happy. Or capable. Stop letting the rest of us down. We're busy and need all the help we can get.

---

1   I've been itching to say this for nearly two decades and finally found a befittingly sardonic way to do so. It's so incredibly cathartic, you have no idea.

DISCLOSURE

First, some housekeeping.

If you can't tell already, this book is not for the faint of heart. If you are easily offended, put it down and walk away. Immediately.

This collection of short stories draws directly from all aspects of my working life. I've worked a lot, from a young age, ascetically juggling multiple roles simultaneously (this I've done always, to this day never having had only one job on the go) and in many different places (and in more than one province)—so please don't make the mistake of assuming anything you are reading is from any one health-care organization in particular. I am confident that any reader will have the imagination to understand that this work, while based on my lived experiences, is a fictional tapestry; as such, any similarities to others' experiences are purely and entirely coincidental.

Naturally, any and all names mentioned in this book are fictitious . . . except for mine. As a registered nurse, I am bound to safeguard privacy, and I have made deliberate and conscientious efforts to do so. This book is about a particular type of health-care environment; any information contained in the following pages should not be a substitute for the medical advice of your health-care professional. Always consult your provider(s) regarding any matter related to your health.

Against the advice of the editors, publisher, and basically everyone, I have not clumped like chapters into thematic sections. I recognize that there are numerous cogent arguments for doing so, but I've simply chosen to ignore them all. Bear with me. First, I don't want readers to skip past anything they don't want to confront or work through (which would have been much easier had themes or specific sections for caregivers, potential residents, and loved ones been neatly batched and laid out), as they would miss out on content they might not otherwise have expected to encounter (and the chance to learn or grow as a result). Shock value is important in making people face difficult and grim realities. You'll learn more this way and come out with a different perspective. Besides, nobody wants to read five sad-sack stories on the trot—let's mix it up. Second, metaphorically speaking, I wanted to inject the type of randomness (manifested in the chapters' order) that mirrors the unpredictable day-to-day experience of how the clinical work tends of unfold. It's a cliché but true: the only thing you can predict is that you can't predict what's going to happen. You can't plan everything out perfectly, and I didn't want this work (again, against sage guidance) to strike the reader as being too polished or romanticized. To make it too slick or sanitized or to glaze over the tough stuff with a thin veneer of stilted language would, to me, be an unrepresentative evasion and an inauthentic depiction of the actual gritty and chaotic nature of the work environment. I wanted to avoid creating a book that was my own version of a generic – and unhelpful – platitude that 'the system is broken'. Sure, there is considerable room for improvement (to be discussed) but there's a lot right with it, too (also addressed) – and for that, we should be grateful. Third, it's my story, and I wanted it to turn out a particular way, unfettered by the discretion of others; I wanted to write an important book—so I chose an important theme. I have driven the process and own the outcomes of my decisions. Besides, it's my name on it, and I'm accountable—for all the good and bad that may come.

In all seriousness, the subject matter of living and working in long-term care can be heavy. Readers are encouraged to check in with how they feel; I recognize that everyone has their own level of tolerance, emotional resilience, and personal lens through which they experience and perceive some of life's most intimate moments and processes. Everyone has a formative past and subsequent paradigm that tend to colour how they see the world—so there's no "right" or "wrong" way to think about this stuff. However, I will admit that I hope the following stories plant a seed or inspire a kernel of an idea that results in reflection, conversation, or deliberate action in the reader. Please delve into the following text with an open mind as you may be inspired to change your opinion and take action.

Warning: while I never intend or mean to offend, I have a natural knack of saying the wrong thing or getting under people's skin—can't help it, I'm afraid. I'm just trying to share the truth as I see it. If you find that my writing style or content elicit strong or unhealthy emotions, please take a break. Even if we think differently, I acknowledge that your feelings and opinions may be legitimate and important; however, as the saying goes: a bomber only gets flak when it's over the target. So, if you're feeling challenged, it's likely an indication of an opportunity for personal growth; in such instances, please choose to adopt an approach of inquisitive curiosity rather than simply to be offended and push back to safeguard long-held beliefs. Moreover, as with most frontline staff, I tend to express duress with profane language; therefore, do not be surprised if it feels like "fuck" is as common in the following text as any form of punctuation. You've been warned.

I should mention also that topics of race, gender, and sexual orientation are woven into the tapestry of this collective narrative because issues around these topics do genuinely crop up. I have chosen to tackle them (albeit in my own way) head-on; I do not believe you can sort-of tell the truth. So, I have written a frank and globally comprehensive account (albeit through my own lens) and that means being honest about everything . . . not just the easy stuff. Ignoring certain topics isn't a solution either. To be absolutely crystal clear, I enjoy working alongside anyone (and everyone) who is competent, reliable, honest, agreeable, and not-entitled—to the exclusion of all other considerations. If you show up reliably, pull your weight, and are well-meaning and collegial, we'll get along just fine.

I'm now in my fourth decade of life. Statistically speaking, there's a good chance that half my life is over. This means that I'm actually closer in age (and certainly in mentality) to those living in long-term care than those in professional schools training for their careers in health care. And I'm finally old enough for people to take me seriously. Whichever, it seemed like an appropriate milestone to take pause, reflect, and write about my career to date.

. . . and even then, I haven't shared nearly half of what I've seen.

TABLE OF CONTENTS

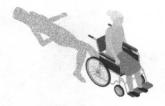

FOREWORD

Thanks for picking up this book. It's a collection of short stories intended to highlight the daily realities of living (and working) in long-term care (LTC). You'll find a handful of chapters informative, while some aspects you might find shocking, some stupefyingly hilarious, and others poignant. All in all, it's an encompassing collection of wild realities.

Not enough is written about life in LTC. The harsh truth is that our society values youth, and little emphasis is placed on life after forty. Moreover, in my experience, even professional schools rarely emphasize LTC or palliative care as legitimate first choices for career paths; they do not garner the type of excitement, glory or respect as emergency, intensive or surgical environments of care. But the secret truth is that long-term care *can be* a "sexy" area of health care in which to work. Stick with this short book until the end, and it'll change your mind. I'm confident that "stodgy" is *not* how you will describe it.

After being surprised continuously by what I'm faced with as a front-line registered nurse (even after working in numerous facilities over nearly two decades in the clinical area of LTC), I wanted to take a stab at sharing how incredulous these stories—and realities—can be.

Paradoxically, they're as personal and individual as they are universal; just change the names and locations and almost anyone should be able to relate to some degree. LTC is worthy of attention and life goes on right until the end.

To date, my career has involved not only front-line work in a handful of different clinical areas (and in different capacities, from being a student working in housekeeping and a nurse on the unit to managing teams and organizations), but also in teaching at the college/ university level and in leading teams both inside and out of health-care environments. It's natural, therefore, that all of these experiences have influenced my perspective and opinions, many of which will be shared throughout (*you've been warned!*). You may not agree with my point of view or chosen tone of delivery—and that's okay; we'll just have to agree to disagree.

If you are not a health-care worker but you know someone who is, *The Wrinkly Ranch* will give some insight into their working lives. I encourage you to talk to them after reading this book, to see if any of these examples have ever happened to them. You may be surprised to find out they'll be able to relate directly . . . *and to think you never knew.*

Working in health care is a 24/7/365.25 commitment, and you see—and participate—in the most intimate and basic human aspects of life. It can take a toll, and there's never an end to the work; no matter how much you do, it's an *infinite* Sisyphean game (i.e., a resident who dies is quickly replaced by another). If you work in health care, this will offer you some healthy cathartic laughter (*don't worry—it's not you who is crazy*). You understand that each day in your line of work is like an unpredictable handful of Nuts n' Bolts—every shift is a whole new ball game.

Similarly, if you know an older adult living in (or soon to live in) LTC, this will offer insight into their daily living experiences and challenges. It will prepare you with reasonable expectations and an ability to better understand and navigate the system. Unfortunately, as we age, life's rites of passage get shittier and shittier; the worst for most is the death of their parents. That's just the nature of it. With any luck, this book may help soften the blow.

I asked myself: *If I wanted to read about this topic, how would I like it to be written?* It would have to feel real, be funny, dark, irreverent (no topic is spared), honest, non-judgmental, and compassionate.

I have chosen to present this material in as unvarnished a manner as possible; as I've stated already, these frankly described stories may not be for the faint of heart. Now, I must emphasize that in no way is the honest or humourous approach of the writing intended to mock this population or take away from any sense of their dignity—quite the opposite, in fact. I contend there is a difference in making light of something serious and not recognizing or appreciating the gravity of that same something serious (no matter *how* serious). I acknowledge that not everyone will share my dark or macabre sense of humour; please recognize that I am not being insensitive but rather coping in the way that works best for me. These stories are based directly on front-line clinical experience and, naturally, have been scrubbed of any/all personal details in order to preserve the confidentiality of residents and staff (i.e., all names that appear are fictitious). Besides, people deserve to be given a transparent account of what goes on. Additionally, in reporting generically, a sense that such stories are experienced universally (and not just in any one particular LTC home) is an underlying theme and central to the lesson I wish to convey.

That said, do not be fooled into thinking that dramatic license or hyperbole have been used liberally in reporting herein. The more unbelievable the story, the more likely it is, in fact, based on lived experience and truth—sometimes, you just can't make up how crazy real life can be. It is because of these incredulous happenings, observations and experiences that I was inspired to reduce them to paper.

Traditionally, this sector of our health-care system has been viewed as "not sexy" to work in, and it rarely gets positive mentions in the media or is seemingly a high priority for recruitment, funding, or investment (well, at least not until something *really* bad happens). However, with the baby boomers marching towards the precipice of requiring LTC beds and given the global pandemic's focus on outbreak management and protecting those most vulnerable, one might hope that greater attention (and permanent funding) will be paid (*finally*) to enhance the global quality of care provided in LTC. Perhaps this book will, in some small way, motivate advocacy and action to such endeavours of improvement.

Last, this book attempts to teach a few things you might not be aware of. It's unapologetically full of all the instructional minutiae that you might not get explained otherwise. As with anything, the devil is in the details. As you might expect, there's death in here—not everyone comes out alive—so, in that respect, it's nearly as entertaining as a murder mystery and a great distraction for an hour or two.

For whatever reason (or concoction of reasons), some people may not wish to hear what really goes on in LTC homes (all the more reason to be told, in my opinion) because, well, ignorance is bliss. As such, the subject has been tabooed for a long time, a real life "sad-bad" that people just avoid talking about, and it's become somewhat controversial. But I disagree with hiding from it. I think facing this topic head-on is a good thing; it's how we ought to interact with the world. We should be present and accepting (even if you're totally gobsmacked, as you may find you are in the scenarios described in the following chapters).

Life can be sad, and some realities are really bad, but the approach of just sweeping this subject under the rug only reinforces and perpetuates taboos by quelling discussion – as if it's a banana peel everyone avoids stepping on. In turn, it only makes it more likely that slippery and "sad-bad" things may continue to happen, as there's no impetus for change. It's a common saying that "to make God laugh, just tell Him/Her your plans"—precisely the same difference between how things "ought" to run and the way things tend to do around The Wrinkly

Ranch. Yet despite everything, great care happens, and life goes on until the end.

So, the residents. The main characters ("characters" being the operative word . . . and that's putting it mildly)—who are these people when you take away the fact that they're old and a lot of their bodies don't function all that well anymore? The often-untold reality is that they can be cranky, rude, racist, and physically aggressive. And smell funny.

Didn't expect that, did you?!

Well, it isn't always harmonious, happy families . . . but as with anyone you spend lots of time with, the residents and staff really do form a big family.

You have to hang out with them long enough to see past the slowness of advanced age, forgetfulness, confusion, deafness, and all the things they can no longer do or are. Even when their defining attributes fade, you see that a person is more than just their physicality. Moreover, by no means are two people alike: some are 'old' at 65 whereas others are 'young' at 90. There is actually more variation in how people present (both physically and mentally) in older adults than at almost any other time in life to the point where you just can't tell how old someone might be. Some people will shock you with how old (or young) they are.

"I know I don't look as handsome as I used to; that's what happens when you're ridden hard and put back wet for 50 years. Sonny, I've had more women than you've had hot dinners!"

You get the idea.

But don't pigeon-hole them or pass judgement too quickly; who they are (still) will surprise you— brief moments of lucidity will reveal surprising aspects of their memory, precious wit, charm, and intelligence—because it's not what you first saw and certainly not what you may have assumed. They were just like you and I are today. They're a window into the past. The subtext is that their stories can be profound and can lend humbling perspective on how trivial our lives' challenges may be. Old people (rather "older adults" in politically correct health-care parlance) need to be loved unconditionally. And so, too, do the people who care for them . . . because they're not perfect, either.

As you read through the pages, remember two things:

1. Getting old happens to everyone. It's the great equalizer.
2. Old people are just that: old, not dead.

Ready? Buckle up and enjoy the ride.

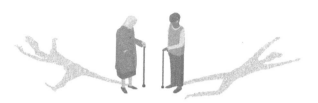

Chapter 1
WHAT'S IN A NAME?

Long-term care. It's in the name: *long*. Like not admitted-and-discharged as quickly as possible. Unlike hospital stays, some residents (in health-care parlance, "patients" are referred to as "residents" because the LTC home is their *home*) will reside for years (some longer than a decade even) in the same facility.

Years. Think about that.

God's Waiting Room, Geezer Glen, Catheter Flats, The Wrinkly Ranch . . . whatever euphemistic pet name you have for long-term care homes, the overall sentiment remains the same: it's the last stop.

But is all hope lost? Is there no joy? Shenanigans? Boondoggles? Great capers? Thefts? Dancing? Laughter? Tears? Sex? (Yeah, you read that right.) If you're a member of the general public, you might be surprised. But if you're a health-care worker, you won't be because nothing surprises you anymore; you've seen everything. And in the off-chance you haven't, you'll believe it. And maybe you will, too, after reading through these stories.

Often, those care providers who enjoy establishing personal relationships with those they serve wind up in in-patient (i.e., longer stay) areas within health care: in-patient mental health, retirement homes, and, of course, long-term care.

As health-care providers, we're bound to treat everyone with respect, care, and dignity—and be in no doubt, that is the case. But, as in real life, even the toughest battle-axe nurse (I can say this because I am one... sometimes) often can't help but be touched by particular residents; everyone has their favourites, even though you're not supposed to. Like the resident who complains incessantly about how bad they think the food is but then asks for seconds. Or the one who always raises their middle finger at you whenever you ask to take their blood sugar and laughs *at you* as they do. Or the one who's mastered their ability to regulate when to pass wind so that it coincides with their tailbone dressing change (and wait until the nurse's face is as close to their ass as possible before farting). And chuckle. Every time.

Nothing to lose and no filter. On either end.

Relationships go both ways: certain residents will always form closer connections to certain members of their care teams than to others. Like with any family member, language becomes familiar, friendly, and generally warmer, abolishing the sterile expectation that everyone must address each other like a member of the Royal Family in a 1950s British television show.

Here's an example:

So, there I am working when I get a call from the nurse on the floor that a resident appears to be having a stroke. They've been found in bed with new slurred speech and one-sided facial drooping—classic, textbook signs. Given their predetermined and agreed-upon level of desired care, an ambulance is called, and they are taken to the hospital forthwith. But not before the following conversation:

Me: *"Hey, Mildred! I've got some good news and bad news. Bad news is that you're having a stroke. Good news is that the nurse caught it quickly, you seem to be recovering, and the ambulance is on its way."*

Several days later (i.e., the next time I'm working), the resident, who has recovered completely and since returned from hospital, is sitting in their favourite spot in front of a computer, playing games and shouts out: *"Hey, bozo! Thanks for saving my life."*

Me: *"Don't mention it . . . but I've regretted it every day since!"*

We both laugh.[2]

----

2   Since time of writing, this resident has passed away. I just happened to be on duty. It was a good death: painless, quick and surrounded by people who cared.

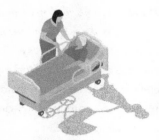

Chapter 2
WHEN IS IT TIME?

There's no obvious or universal predetermined trigger that lets the world know that it's time to be admitted to LTC. No flashing lights, chiming bells, or whistles blown. Interestingly, it's often quite the opposite: more a gradual, insidious, and pernicious decline in function that is visible only in retrospect. This means that vigilance is particularly important.

What's worse is that some older adults are really quite skilled at faking being completely lucid when they are not (I can see the irony and foreshadowing here, as this will most likely be me . . . to a T). Additionally, they may be resistive even to the idea of entering any environment of organized care. This only makes a difficult time harder. Nothing is easy.

The risks of putting off the decision too long are real. Without constant supervision or assistance, grave and common consequences such as falling and breaking a hip, under- or overdosing on medication, wandering outside during periods of extreme weather, or leaving something on that results in a fire hazard, may result. Moreover, the risks of less urgent but equally serious declines in hygiene or nutrition, which tend to correlate positively with increased confusion, ought not to be overlooked either.

If you are involved in or responsible for the care of an older adult, it's best to be proactive and dispassionate. Find out how the admission process works in your area well ahead of time. This will give you an informed idea of what the local criteria are to qualify for a long-term care bed and any costs involved. You might be surprised to learn that there's a considerable waitlist . . . good thing you thought to get in early then (because what you don't want is to realize suddenly you need one and then be new on the list). While beds are distributed according to acuity of need, there may be room to honour a family's preference for a bed in a particular home (i.e., for reasons of geographic proximity). While efforts are made to respect a first, second, or third choice, a family may have to face the possibility of taking the first bed that becomes available, albeit one that was not on their preferred list.

Many stay-at-home options exist, wherein caring help comes to visit at regular intervals (for prescribed tasks). They are absolutely viable and appropriate for a while, but they may not be sufficiently comprehensive as an end-game strategy if a person's ability to function continues to decline. If at-home support is in place for an older adult, it's always best to keep in touch with them to gauge when the time for more support with increased frequency has arrived.

Generally speaking, long-term care is the appropriate venue of care for older adults who are no longer able to care for themselves, due to either physical or mental decline. Naturally, there are exceptions, but the overall premise is that those admitted can no longer live independently in a safe manner, as to do so would present a danger to themselves. There really isn't any difference in the admission process between males and females other than most facilities will not group a male and a female together in a room unless they are spouses (and, even then, sometimes they aren't . . . by mutual request).

On the upside, it's interesting to witness (and it's not uncommon) newly admitted residents be pleasantly surprised at the unexpected positives of entering a home. Regular hot baths are usually at the top of the list, followed by decreased stress in not having to worry about pesky meal prep, medication administration, and other daily chores. Help with being toileted (i.e., not having to sit in soiled clothing or bedding) and being able to socialize (or not—totally up to individual preference) are other positive healthy outcomes that promote dignity, higher quality care, and enjoyment of life—all in a safe environment that's monitored 24/7.

These advantages should be emphasized, as what's the value of being independent when you can't do anything good on your own?! Put your feet up, and let others do the work—you've earned it.

It's time.

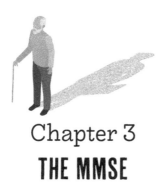

Chapter 3
THE MMSE

The Mini-Mental State Exam (MMSE)—it's a simple conversational test, scored out of thirty points, that's used to establish a rough overall picture of the baseline state of a resident's memory and capacity to execute simple tasks and follow direction. Specifically, it asks questions to test short-and longer-term memory recall, ability to follow direction, fine motor skills, basic math skills, oral comprehension, language skills, and spatial awareness. All questions are simple and straightforward, yet the differences in test scores highlight any underlying deficiencies very quickly. In some cases, it is only with such a process that those who seem with-it conversationally reveal just how confused and unable to cope they truly are.

Typically, these tests are completed with a resident prior to placement in long-term care (i.e., cognitively speaking, how urgently do they need twenty-four-hour supervision and care?) and every so often once admitted. A repeat test is usually administered to confirm that they are receiving the most appropriate level of care *vis-à-vis* their ability to remain their own primary decision-maker (or if a substitute decision-maker, a power of attorney, is required due to lack of mental competence). It is particularly helpful at distinguishing between perceived and actual ability to function well cognitively—and these results can be surprising. Cognitive ability isn't binary, and lines can become blurred quite easily.

For example, one resident, who had worked in the emergency services for years, was mistaken at front reception for a visitor given how well they presented physically (i.e., they were strong and could walk well independently). However, later that same day, they were found at the front once again, trying to get out because they had seen "their team" practising scaling the building (a visual hallucination). Later that evening, when they were being assisted, the personal support worker (PSW) found that they had placed their wallet in their "back pocket" (i.e., in their briefs) as they had planned to be out that day.

The registered nurse (RN) is typically the one responsible for sitting with residents to run through these tests. The process is always revealing and can be very insightful and an enjoyable experience to learn about the resident in question—most of the time.

Many appreciate the fact that someone is actually sitting down to have a conversation with them, for no apparent reason, that doesn't seem to be rushed or in which they are required simply to process the next item (even though it really is). Accordingly, the opportunity to speak with someone usually results in long-winded conversations, strolling down memory lane, wherein the RN tries to keep them on track (not that Burt's cottage in '55 wasn't a great place to be that summer).

Now . . . where was I? Oh yeah.

The answers are always revealing. As you might expect, those who were engineers for thirty-five years can't put two words together (let alone spell anything correctly) but can whiz through the math and spatial awareness drawings more quickly and accurately than half the current staff. Others can follow the oral direction to a T but can't remember what was asked of them two minutes ago. They may, however, have no problem discussing in great detail how they survived being bombed out of their home *twice* in London during the Blitz, managing to survive only by hiding under the stairs (!), but when asked what the date is, the best they can reply is, *"I don't know ... winter 1978?"*

Perhaps the most telling aspect of the test—demonstrating the resident's current state of mind— comes towards the end when they are asked to write a sentence. It can be about anything. More often than you might think (or perhaps simply as a reaction specific to this writer), they write:

"Fuck off!"

The inclusion of the exclamation point highlights correct punctuation given the use of imperative verb tense. Full points for that one. Brevity is the soul of wit, after all.

Nobody likes to waste time being pestered with silly questions. Not even old people.

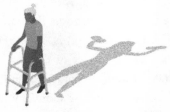

Chapter 4

STUFF FAMILIES SHOULD KNOW

(WHEN YOU'VE GOT A LOVED ONE IN LTC)

When the day finally comes that a family gets word there is a bed available in a long-term care home (albeit perhaps not at their first—or second—choice of home), the admission and move-in process begins. Honestly, though, you should take the first bed that becomes available; don't keep waiting for "the perfect bed" at your (arbitrary) first home of choice.

Think of it as moving back into a college/university residence, although slightly less fun (the "exams" are far more unpleasant this time) but with a greater chance of being mooned by your peers. Gotta take the rough with the smooth. Choose to be excited.

Despite the natural angst of getting to know a new environment and people, most residents (and their families) are actually relieved and experience an *improvement* in their quality of their lives. For example, with all the mechanical lifts and specialized tubs, residents can once again enjoy a hot bath or shower, and families do not have to stress or worry (or be physically exhausted) regarding their loved one's care needs being met. They are. Some new residents are thrilled to move in just so that they can get away from an abusive spouse, family member or to escape substandard living conditions. Sad but true. Others appreciate being able to participate easily in societal rights like voting in elections. Indeed, the improvements in their mood and confidence are so encouraging to behold once they realize they are free to make friends and have important social interactions—no more being lonely, isolated, hungry, dirty and fearful living alone. For these reasons (and many others besides), long-term care homes should never be regarded as a punishment – but quite the opposite.

Unfortunately, during the admission process, not everything that ought to be shared is communicated clearly (i.e., the daily nuts and bolts). If you have someone in LTC, perhaps you might benefit from knowing the following information (and if so, kindly consider making adjustments accordingly):

- **Be informed:** Be prepared to share what your resident's medical conditions are. What medications they are on. Who their (previous) physician(s) is. What their allergies are. Bring their health card and any relevant insurance documents that outline drug coverage. Basically, anything and everything that will need to be passed along to clarify their history, needs, and preferences.

- **Be an advocate:** Staff truly appreciate that you advocate for your loved one (it's far more preferable than in cases where the families are impossible to contact and never around). Establish a good working relationship with the full-time nursing team; make it easy for them to reach out. Trust is established with all those back-and-forth conversations. If everyone is on the same page and singing from the same song sheet, the resident only stands to benefit from this symbiosis when quick decisions need to be made. The best way to remain actively involved in a resident's life is by cultivating a healthy, respectful rapport with the staff; learning to lean on each other is the best approach.

However, please don't pester the staff—it only slows them down. In fact (and admittedly rather selfishly), one of few benefits of an illness outbreak being declared is that family access is then restricted; consequently, staff can focus on providing care with fewer distractions or interruptions. Visiting hours do exist for a reason. By pestering, we mean to ask that you not call the nurse ten times a day (and especially not to have your mom's pillow fluffed—seriously).

- **Be patient:** Please learn to be especially patient and understanding; it's a 24/7/365.25 enterprise, and you can't always expect (or request) that only certain staff care for your parent. To say that the staff are faced with competing demands is an understatement. They're doing their level best. Kindly learn when shift changes and mealtimes occur and be mindful to avoid calling, whenever possible, at these especially busy times. Conversely, never – *ever* – remark that it is 'quiet'. To the staff, this comment is no different than fingers nails on a chalk board; anytime anyone ever says it's 'quiet' you've then jinxed it and chaos on the unit will quickly ensue. Please and thank you.

- **Label and limit:** Label everything but still expect that things will go missing. Limit any valuables left on-site. Most importantly, don't ram-jam their rooms full of stuff; less is more (and far safer). Mechanical lifts, stretchers, walkers, and wheelchairs need room to manoeuvre safely. This is just as much for the staff as it is for the residents themselves— nobody needs more tripping hazards. Think of it this way as well: you want to leave the room in such a way that it will be as easy to clean (and clean thoroughly) as possible.

- **Check in first:** When your parent complains, please check in with the care team before starting to worry. Recognize that what you are being told by your mom/dad might best be taken with a grain of salt. Use it as a jumping-off point for a conversation, rather than gospel from which to launch into worry, concern, or an entirely unjustified tirade of verbal abuse directed towards the staff. Again, trust is everything; work together.

- **Say no to accessories:** Wearing jewelry is never advisable. Risk of loss/theft aside, rings will cause problems and will lose their "perfect" fit. If someone is retaining fluid and swells, a ring may need to be cut in order to be removed, and even then, it might cause the skin to tear. (One resident fell and got their ring finger caught in a door jam and was unable to pull it free. The otherwise preventable tissue damage resulted in the finger being amputated.)

  Also, do not give your mom/grandmother metal hair clips. If they fall and hit their head, those clips will impale and tear their skin. Nothing is as traumatic as having to wash the blood from a head wound or having to shave their hair around the injury site in order for a dressing to be applied.

- **Be mindful:** If you are setting up a TV or computer, make everything as simple as possible and make concerted efforts to tie or tape down any cords. Again, think about minimizing tripping hazards wherever possible. If in a room that is shared with another resident, please be cognizant that the staff may not be able to monitor the volumes of competing TVs constantly. (Just because you want to speak to your resident on the phone, you can't expect your conversation to come at the expense of the other resident either leaving the room or turning off their TV). Consider buying your resident (and perhaps their roommate too) headphones; give the gift of silent, private enjoyment of their TV, radio, or phone call. Besides, it's tough to put a price on maintaining friendly relations and the ability to sleep when in a small, shared space.

- **Be thoughtful:** Some especially thoughtful things you can do include paying for a subscription to your loved one's favourite newspaper, magazine, audiobook platform, or TV channels. Have fresh flowers (a *small* bouquet) delivered. When you visit, bring them a nice coffee from the outside world. Bring in the family pet. Take them out for a drive. Ask for their advice on matters of seeming "importance" in your current life—no doubt they'll be able to offer a sobering perspective.

And that's it, really. Perspective is everything, after all.

Looking back, living in "rez" college or university is often among the best part of life, and with a chance at a second act, who wouldn't want to go out having a blast?!

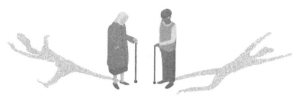

Chapter 5
IT'S A BIG PLACE

(AND HAS MORE BEDS THAN MOST SMALL HOSPITALS)

Most don't realize how large long-term care homes can be. With newer homes especially, they can have more in-patient beds than small hospitals (we're talking close to 200 beds), spanning across multiple floors, units, and wings—it takes a while to walk from one end to the other.

At least those few residents still interested in keeping fit can get in a good long stroll with their walkers after breakfast (and yes, impromptu walker races have been known to occur).

While every home is different, larger ones consist of similar attributes: long hallways with rooms on either side for resident bedrooms, communal tub/shower rooms, clean and dirty laundry, garbage, supplies, and a nursing station. There is usually a large communal dining room, as well as a couple of common area rooms for group activities or watching TV.

Everywhere is brightly lit, and there are handrails along the walls on either side of common areas. If beige—in all its hues and shades—is your favourite colour, then you're in for a treat; there's a symphony of the stuff on most vertical surfaces, broken up only by the artwork hung on the walls (artwork, which by the way, is placed too high for anyone sitting in a wheelchair to look at properly?!). Outside the door to each bedroom, there are often little enclosed glass "memory" boxes for each resident to place a handful of their chosen memorabilia, adding a personal touch.

There are generally large metal doors (to comply with fire regulations perhaps?) at either end of each unit, which, when in an outbreak, help enforce isolation measures (for some reason, they always make me think of the water-tight doors on the Titanic—these seem just as useless).

In a busy shift, staff can cover seven or eight kilometres of walking. Easily. And that's assuming a full staffing complement; if units are running short of personnel, the distance covered per person rises disproportionally with the ensuing chaos. One PSW, on a sixteen-hour day, clocked almost twenty kilometres of walking—before having eight hours off, only to return to do it all again.

The building itself is like another character in the plot of daily living. Is it too hot? Too cold? (It usually falls on the RN to record ambient indoor temperatures—not that anyone really ever looks at this log.) Is something not working? (A resident's phone and TV cable lines are frequent annoyances.) Too bright? Too dark? Too smelly? Too wet? Can't find something (or someone)? Where's the best place to hide these extra supplies? How can I fit into this room with the mechanical lift? Why is the staff washroom so far away? Why does the resident shower on the second floor run cold when the janitor's closet tap on the first floor isn't properly shut off?!

Getting to know the nuances of the building itself (e.g., when the best time is to start the second round of baths and showers so there's enough hot water) is often part of the most valuable (albeit unrecognized) organizational knowledge staff acquire as they gain experience.

With up to thirty residents to any given unit, the natural logistics of time and distance can't help but influence the where/when/how care is provided. Being in outbreak (with having to don a fresh gown, pair of gloves, and a mask between each resident) only slows progress and can alter the order of operations. Only by understanding the physical layout of a unit can one start to understand why, when a resident rings for assistance, it can take time for staff to respond. To be clear, the staff do their best, but in a six-to-one, eight-to-one, or ten-one ratio of residents per staff, it can be impossible to meet everyone's needs simultaneously. A call to 911 for fire crew to arrive could reasonably be expected to result in a faster response time than some residents can expect from busy PSWs. This isn't anyone's fault—it is truly the system's problem.

This is how things go sideways . . . easily. It's simply a numbers game.

This issue means people are rushed, which means staff can't spend as much time with residents as they may otherwise wish to, which means workarounds are often implemented, even if unofficially (e.g., stashing supplies). I am not condoning these types of strategies or behaviours; rather, I am simply explaining root causes while admitting we can all do better. Fundamentally, this might be the underlying reason why homes may struggle to provide care much beyond the necessities of life at times: everything is run as efficiently as possible and resources are limited.

For example, staff are a limited resource (either for reasons of funding or availability); when a unit is running short, the few have the same amount of work to complete (and in the same amount of time). This is how a resident's incontinence can lead quickly to skin breakdown; not everyone in a wet chair or bed, briefs, or clothes can get changed and cleaned right away. It's difficult for the body's wounds to heal if nutritional and protein levels are low—which they almost always are if residents don't eat sufficient armounts. And who would if the sustenance is unidentifiable, served sloppy, minced, pureed . . . and cold?

Sometimes, the thinking behind what's placed where is baffling and defies any logic relating to good ergonomics. All you want when you're so busy is for commonly used items to fall to hand— but that's too much to ask. Take, for example, the placement of towel dispensers (the type with the paper roll inside that you're simply supposed to pull on but end up having to roll from the knob on the side) as a perfect illustration of something poorly thought-out. Somehow, they manage to find themselves bolted to the wall so close to a corner as to require the user to contort their fingers simply to rotate the wheel. Or, a personal favourite, when the placement of the tiny bar fridge in the med room is nestled under the counter and in the corner . . . with the door opening the wrong way (i.e., in front of you, not against the wall). Once you've leaned in to reach over and down, you proceed to hit your funny bone (because you're now boxed in by the radiator that protrudes from the wall), which causes you to drop the vial of medication you went in to get in the first place. I won't go into the elaborate process that is then required to document the wastage and reordering of this medication.

It's also interesting how buildings were not designed with basic health-care considerations in mind. Take, for example, the rather inconvenient need to be able to remove a dead body discreetly. Unfortunately, there's no way to wheel out the gurney without having to roll it past at least one dining room or common gathering area.

And who doesn't want a harsh reminder of what's waiting for them interrupting their enjoyment of a cold, minced, pureed meal while sitting in a wet brief?

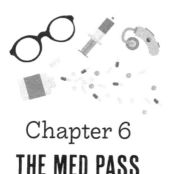

Chapter 6
THE MED PASS

In any health-care facility, there is a tremendous array of different types of professional and supportive staff on hand (and on call) at any given time. When you consider that such buildings must be populated by the appropriate workers 24/7/365.25, you start to understand the scope of the logistical challenge involved in making sure the right people show up (to the right places) in the right numbers and at the right times. Think of a tightly wound mechanical watch: one cog missing, broken, or out-of-step, and stuff starts to go downhill fast (although even a broken clock is right twice a day, but I digress . . .).

The vast majority of the hands-on care (changing, clothing, bathing, feeding, etc.) is the responsibility of the personal support workers (PSWs). They're the real heroes (more on them later) who bare the physical brunt of the acts of caring. Depending on the time of day, there ought to be two to four PSWs working on a unit of twenty to thirty (or more) residents. A registered practical nurse (RPN) often leads the team of PSWs and is the go-to person in charge of any particular unit (i.e., one RPN per unit). They are responsible for the majority of the treatments, provision of medication, and assessments. The registered nurse (RN) usually takes on a supervisory role and steps in to provide additional consultative and hands-on clinical support for the PSW and RPN teams. Complex treatments and advanced assessments will also fall to the RNs. Finally, nurse practitioners (NPs) and physicians (MDs) are available for diagnostic and prescriptive consultative support.

As one might imagine, it takes an incredible amount of organization to provide the necessary attention to roughly thirty people every day—particularly when it comes to ensuring the right medications are provided (in the right form and dose) to each resident on time—all while real life happens and distracts you from the task at hand (think: call bells, phone calls, people falling, being asked questions, working short—you get the idea). Indeed, nursing is not for those who cannot multitask or work quickly under the gun.

The nurse on the unit will usually have a large five- or six-drawer cart on wheels, with various pull-out table surfaces and other appendages, that contains all the necessary medications for the residents (picture one of those large industrial toolboxes on wheels; that's the size). If people only knew that these rather innocent-looking "crates" contained residents' jewellery and money, narcotics, alcohol, CBD oil, and lubricants, they might start to wonder: *What's really going on, here?*

The "med pass" is the anchor task for the nurse on the unit. Depending on the shift (i.e., days, afternoons, or nights), it can happen multiple times within their period of responsibility. Most medication coincides with mealtimes (because who doesn't want an amuse-bouche of eleven pills crushed and mixed in a foul-tasting applesauce cocktail with some oily laxative to wash it down?!), but it's not uncommon for residents to be prescribed medication that is to be given every one-to-two hours . . . around the clock.

And that's assuming the people are easy to find—but old people aren't always where you last left them. They do tend to wander about, after all. When that happens, you have to find them before you can give them what they need. In a really large building. And this assumes both that you know who you are looking for and who you find is actually the who you are looking for. For example, if a resident's name is Don but, for whatever reason, Don prefers to go by Jack and there are two other "real" Jacks on the same unit (who both go by their actual name), a new staff member ensnared in an unfamiliar unit has their work cut out to disentangle that potential morass. The last thing you want to do is give one resident another's medication . . . all because of a simple misunderstanding based on a shared name. Moreover, residents' appearances change over time, so they might not always resemble their own picture from the time of admission. See how confusing and time consuming this can be (never mind trying to find them along a long hallway with over twenty rooms)? Seriously.

How would you like to be woken up at 6:00 a.m. every day to the following transactional quid pro quo?

"Happy Sunday! Let's start your day off right . . . with some narcotics!"

"Am I crazy? Why am I here?"

"No, you're not crazy . . . you're just old. You're ninety-eight."

"Oh, so that's why I'm feeling upside-down and back-to-front."

No amount of formal post-secondary education makes it easier (or the provider more skilled) at ensuring a morning med pass for thirty-odd residents—that can include over 225 medications (actually a *conservative estimate*) to be completed perfectly without a single error within two hours (just in time for the next one to start). Remember, these 225 medications come in different forms: puffers, pills (whole, broken-in-two, or crushed? In applesauce or chocolate pudding?), patches, insulins, eye drops, ear drops, IVs, hearing aids, bowel regimen, and so on. The *expectation* is to not make a single mistake . . . all while your phone is going off and you have countless other interruptions (one thing happens, and your day can be thrown off entirely). As other professions have been described, nursing can be both "impossible and extremely difficult" – where you anticipate that despite all efforts, results will be "unsatisfying".

Oh, and after the five minutes it takes to prep everything

(double-checking what's ordered with what you have been provided to give, then crushing all the pills and mixing them in applesauce), the resident refuses to take their cocktail of medications or takes everything only to spit it all out... because it tastes awful. And who can blame them, really?

One extreme example was highlighted by a "responsive" resident (i.e., aggressive) who threw (thankfully, now cold) coffee into the face of a dietary worker. The resident in question would accept meds only when they were crushed up and mixed in their coffee (a preference based on a habit formed before admission to LTC). See the problem?

In fact, it's not uncommon for residents to refuse to take their medications which only exacerbates underlying conditions and makes fighting infections all the more challenging. Ensuring medications are taken properly is particularly difficult when residents demonstrate paranoia and are convinced you are trying to poison or kill them with their medications. Patience is a virtue, indeed.

The irony is that residents can be more interested and concerned (jealous, even) in others' medications than they are their own (... *maybe THAT will help my bowels move?!*). Explaining why you can't play 'tradesies' between residents who want to swap meds (i.e.: narcotics, sedatives, antibiotics, psychiatric, heart or bowel meds, etc.) can take a while.

To counter this point, I once had an elderly gentleman explain the following: "Young man (meanwhile, I was in my mid-30s), if you'd give her a big wet kiss, what's the difference whether you eat her sandwich, drink her tea or have one of her pills?"

Touché.

When handing out medications, the need to supervise to prevent accidental ingestion of other's medication regimens is real and unrelenting.

If residents, however pleasant, "cute," or innocent looking, can't be trusted to take their pills independently—because they'll end up hidden in plant pots, in a hanky in the garbage, in a night table (not necessarily theirs), or in their pillowcase—why fight it? Insanity may be defined as repeating a task in an identical manner while expecting a different result.

. . . and is it *really* necessary to prescribe *so* many medications?! What's the real goal here: Simply to prolong life or to maintain the highest quality of life for the most reasonable amount of natural time remaining?! Great point for all advocates to consider when discussing the type of care their loved one ought to receive.

Also to be considered is that not every nurse conducting a med pass is actually familiar with the needs, preferences, and prescriptions of every resident. Therefore, additional time is often needed to complete the due diligence required to ensure that each medication, route, and dose prescribed are all present, correct and appropriate (sometimes, the high volume of narcotics and/or insulins would OD most people— *try taking eighty units of insulin*). So, now it's a rush against the clock because you want to finish in time to start the next pass as scheduled.

Never mind all the dressing changes, wound and skin care, and other scheduled assessments.

The term "warehousing" often applies to the rudimentary, task-focused type of care that is traditionally associated with long-term care. There is no more fitting an example than simply going from resident to resident (in a hurry) to give them their pills. No time to entertain anything but the most superficial conversation. No time to dilly-dally. Even when you know all they really want is to talk to someone. Tough stuff—and that can wear on the staff.

In loose terms, moral distress refers to when someone cannot act as they believe they should given the pressures and/or challenges placed upon them. Not being able to meet every resident's needs is distressing to conscientious clinical staff (who feel both helpless and guilty despite devoting their best efforts) – and you wonder why so many nurses are leaving the profession.

It goes without saying that no nurse responsible for a med pass has any problem fitting in their 10,000 steps a day. Or 15,000.

Just ask one.

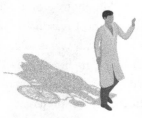

Chapter 7

THE ROLE OF MANAGEMENT AND LEADERSHIP

I can imagine a few managers and executive leaders leaning forward ever so awkwardly as their eyes catch glimpse of this chapter. Fear not. Effective leaders at all levels are vital—not only for ensuring execution of important and strategic items but for setting the tone within an organization. Also, it must be said from the outset that very few fields, short of nuclear power, are as highly regulated as LTC; to say leaders have their work cut out for them to navigate and fulfill all requirements is a colossal understatement. This point alone anchors my respect for anyone in a position of leadership in LTC today.

I view the role of a leader as one of setting and communicating important, strategic direction and priorities made in the best interests of an organization, consistent with its mission, vision, and values. They guide and communicate the distillation of priorities to the absolutely essential; if you claim to have ten, you have none. It is about being strategic and effective without playing politics. It is important that leaders offer clarity by setting performance targets and outlining the processes and metrics upon which achievement will be evaluated. Remember: *what gets measured, gets managed.* Creating the necessary framework of policies and procedures while holding people accountable (through transparent and understood performance management and conflict resolution processes) are essential to guarantee a level playing field and to ensure compliance to all requisite standards. Metaphorically speaking, the decision of which wall to place a ladder falls to the (executive) leader, the role of a manager would be to determine how best to secure that ladder on said wall and ensure their team executes the leader's vision as intended, to the standards set. Front-line workers are accountable for completing the work assigned to them competently and in a manner consistent with the guiding instructions, policies, procedures, and accepted best practices. Everyone should comport themselves unpretentiously and in a manner consistent with the values of the organization.

Great leadership is really rather rare. It transcends the role and serves by building, providing, and multiplying value through virtuous, ethical decisions and actions. It is to be a calm, reassuring hand at the wheel during turbulent and uncertain times. It is to listen to others in a humble and reflective manner. It is to create a safe, non-judgmental space where people can fail without fear of reprisal; in so doing, to build engagement and to unlock the latent capacity of those who are disengaged and disenchanted. If, as a leader, you can demonstrate forgiveness and leave room for well-intended employees to flounder as they learn, self-correct and grow, you might find that not only do they more than make up for themselves but become steadfast in their devotion to you, their team and to the organization. Courage stems from trust. Truly, leaving room for redemption by seeing the good and providing space and time is, in my opinion, an under-utilized leadership strategy and approach to management.

By being at once both externally and internally focused, leaders foster relationships and drive engagement equally with community stakeholders and partnering providers as they might among the internal workforce. It is to set expectations, hire and promote staff and invest the time to groom new leaders (including their replacement) such that the organization continues to operate smoothly upon their departure. It is to provide the tools and resources necessary... and then to get out of the way. In so doing, their legacy is evident in the sustained prosperity and reputation of the organization over the short, medium, and longer horizons.

I've held roles at all levels, been witness to excellence . . . and what not to do. In equal measure. I've tried to soak it all up and never be too proud to learn, adapt, and improve. I believe that my track record of continuous education speaks to this commitment. My approach has always been to treat everyone the same and to be fair, patient, and kind while tackling any issue at hand in a non-personal way. For example, before rampaging to any conclusions, I try to ask myself why a reasonable person would do X; sometimes slowing down works as well as charging full steam ahead. In my experience, rarely does a knee-jerk reaction lead to positive outcomes. Often, with respect to a suboptimal choice or judgment taken by a direct report, I ask first how I might have contributed and, consequently, if they were unknowing, unable, or unwilling before deciding on the most appropriate approach to address the situation. That said, I know I'm far from perfect and that my style of leadership does not work for everyone.

In my experience, leadership is much like family, in that everyone will have their own unique interpretation of what it means and what their preferences are; not everyone likes to be led in the same manner, and not all approaches work equally well with everyone. To be most effective, you need to have a flexible approach and expect to adjust according to the situation and people involved.

It can be frustrating to witness the damage caused when someone in a leadership position chooses a disproportionately harsh approach or focuses myopically on today to the detriment of a healthy future relationship with a reporting staff or colleague. Word soon gets out of any perceived mistreatment and it's then very difficult to re-establish collegial working relationships. Not much of a staff retention (or recruitment) strategy. In fact, very little is more damaging or condescending than a leader sounding magnanimous for simply offering the very support to those on the front line that they ought to by very definition of their role. Indeed, a judicious leader needs to be able to see past the end of their nose. However, it must be noted that the pendulum swings too far the other way as well: the revolving door of those in leadership positions carries its own cocktail of deleterious consequences for their team and organization. For example, if leaders are replaced every one-to-two years, staff recognize this pattern quickly; consequently, why should anyone listen to – much less change for – someone who is effectively disposable and will likely be gone in the near future!? What a disincentive to apply (much less aspire to) to vacant leadership positions – hence the dearth of quality applicants. Speak to any veteran front-line staff and it's highly likely that they'll have lost count of the number of managers and leaders who have come and gone since their arrival. It is my view that for meaningful change to take hold in any organization, everyone needs to be supported and accepted as imperfect – including leaders. Without unshakable, kind personal support, understanding, professional coaching and time to adapt and improve over the longer term, nobody can be expected to master their role, much less make headway in moving the needle forward.

And remember to be patient: progress isn't always linear (even with a low-pass filter).

Speaking of change, we ought to address the issue of effective change management; leaders driving change lose people when transitions are implemented too quickly, seemingly randomly, without collective buy-in or even understandable and reasonable rationale. The most competent leaders guide change in such a way as to engage the greatest number of people directly involved, throughout the entire process, so much so that they believe they drove the process themselves and own and embrace the outcomes. In my view, these are very real challenges everywhere, but perhaps most especially in LTC. Clear, consistent and repeated communication are essential; once you've communicated, you then need to repeat yourself. Again and again.

Within the sphere of LTC, leaders are accountable for ensuring the home meets the myriad of Ministry standards and requisite reporting. Those in the leadership team are the first point of contact on behalf of the home for all community partners and stakeholders. Financial demands must be met and juggled with the daily turnover of communication and education with residents, families, and staff. In privately owned homes, financial accountability and reporting to boards must be an unenviable duty. Staffing the building is a full-time role in itself—not only filling the gaps but managing performance, turnover, and hiring adequately. Maintaining stability in the workplace is often overlooked and certainly underrated.

Staff appreciate recognition, considered and informed individual praise, and being inspired of the meaningfulness of their work that's often forgotten among the demands of the daily grind. This common revelation fosters a culture where you grow closer to your colleagues and thereby cultivate a sense of shared responsibility.

A quick note here to underline the importance of the role played by informal leaders: anyone can choose to be a leader in their attitudes, mindset, conversation, and actions. It's incredible to see the positive difference in the working environment when people go out of their way to be helpful and generous. It's contagious.

Ultimately, the role of leaders is no different than running a large-sized business: you are responsible for everything 24/7/365.25 (yes, that means being on call, too). Like the rest of us, they're just normal people doing their best, given all the demands and pressures placed upon them.

They deserve to be given credit and afforded forgiveness, too.[3]

---

3   While I've long been an advocate for thanking staff to recognize their efforts, it must be said that it's far rarer for a staff member to thank their boss, manager, leader, or directing executive. Just wanted to point that out. You might owe your job to their efforts – *on ne sait jamais*. They are overworked and under-paid, too.

Chapter 8
MAINTENANCE

With any institutionally sized building—and all the industrial systems within that are required to make the place function—some of the most under-recognized crews work in maintenance.

These are the guys (and gals) who work in the unseen underworld to make sure the building and equipment work properly 24/7 (that's right, they're on call too). They know the building inside-out with all its esoteric quirks and features.

. . . like if the water in the second-floor shower room isn't warm enough, double-check to see if the janitor's closet's tap on the first floor isn't dripping.

Doesn't make intuitive sense to me, either. But they aren't wrong. Problem solved. Glad I asked.

And they're always just the nicest, most helpful, down-to-earth types—so patient with everyone forever asking something of them (they must think people are useless and can't do anything themselves . . . but never let on).

Inexhaustible patience must rank among the most important qualities in successful candidates for any position in maintenance. How else could they work happily while always being interrupted, having to step aside to let people by constantly, redoing what they just did recently (because it's been redamaged for the zillionth time), or re-explaining the most basic things to those not mechanically minded? Remember, they're accountable all while adhering to a budget that's never sufficient to be both adequate in the moment and forward-thinking. Being innovative on a shoestring often results in just getting by. Hence why the A/C always seems to give up the ghost during the first heat wave every summer.

Working hand-in-glove (pardon any pun) with housekeeping/environmental services, a myriad of behind-the-scenes services are completed simply to support the clinical staff so that they can perform the care that's required.

From making sure back-up generators function properly (and explaining how the monthly test goes . . . every month . . . to everyone; same with fire drills, by the way) to fixing furniture and equipment (and removing anything that could be even remotely unsafe) to painting the walls and patching the drywall on a daily basis (just to keep up with the constant scuffs and holes created by carts and scooters), maintenance crews can never find enough hours in the day to ensure the home looks pristine and everything is working perfectly.

They deserve a gold medal when having to tolerate the clinical staff stumbling to explain what's wrong with a piece of equipment as they can't help themselves from giggling throughout (i.e., "The sit-stand lift's legs won't close; they're open all the way. . . but it'll still go up-and-down just fine. How promiscuous!").

Interestingly, painting is always going on somewhere (every time a resident passes away, their room is given a thorough clean and freshening). It's astounding to see just how many shades of beige are available.

Also, there's no point in removing old wallpaper . . . just paint over it. Multiple times.

(Ever wonder how many coats of paint it would take to enclose an entire room? Well, it has to be more than your first guess because even after twenty coats, there doesn't seem to be much change.)

The need to provide a safe environment (beyond just controlling the seasonally adjusted ambient temperature) governs many aspects of their responsibilities. For example, making sure water temperatures are kept within normal limits (i.e., not too hot) is important because you need to be mindful that frail, thin skin scalds particularly easily. Ensuring all fire-related detection, containment and suppression safety systems are working well (and devising approved anti-tampering devices on all fire station pulls to stop false alarms from residents who, confused or otherwise, pull on them) is another example. Testing and maintaining the proper, safe function of all lifts, mechanical beds and bathtubs are other examples that highlight the types of responsibilities that fall to this group. Ensuring all mechanised lifting equipment is in proper working order safeguards not only the residents but the staff; without lifts, strain injuries (particularly of the back) would be far more common – and nobody should have to be worried about their physical safety when going into work.

Further to the example of mechanical beds, ensuring proper func-tion means more than just testing the up-and-down motors repeat-edly; testing that a resident can't slide and get caught between the rails or head/foot boards is vital, too. Anything to prevent falls and skin tears (not to mention staff musculoskeletal injuries) is a must. Preventing even one negative outcome often saves more than the crew is paid. For a week. Never mind the pain, discomfort, or suffering that's also prevented.

Other safety measures the maintenance crews take care of include lighting— having to ensure common areas meet minimum brightness standards (measured in lumens), fixing blown fuses (which happen all the time whenever people try to plug in six things in one socket . . . typically the borderline hoarders), and making sure the elevators work properly (and it isn't easy to keep the stopping heights on each floor calibrated perfectly to enable people to roll in and out without a hump).

Another insightful tidbit about their job: they must be asked to unclog at least one toilet every day.

Don't ask.

. . . and please mind the walls; they've been freshly painted.

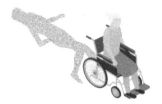

Chapter 9
NO A/C AND WRINKLY RANCHISMS

It feels like every summer, it's the same thing: as if, on cue, during the first head-wave (i.e., 30° Celsius plus humidity, making it feel almost 40), the air conditioning breaks. Every. Single. Year. It's disgusting and exhausting to work in; you're drenched in sweat. For hours. Not to mention, any urinary or fecal odours seem to be rendered that much more pungent as a result. Utterly delightful.

Thought: When a baby is wet, you change them, but when you're a health-care worker, you get to wear wet clothes for eight to twelve (or sixteen) hours. Interesting, no? (Good thing you're not reading this in smell-e-vision, eh?! Certainly would singe the nostrils). Nobody likes swamp ass (aka 'swass'), *swalls, swoob* (aka 'mountain dew'), or *swussy* (no need to spell it out what any of those mean). It can feel like an eight-hour trip to a sweat lodge (atoning for anything, are we?!).

It's never fun to sweat like a whore in church.

When you sweat that much, it can feel like your forehead has sprung a leak, and it just won't stop. The salt stings your eyes. Other than trying to consume your own body weight in fluids to try and remain adequately hydrated, one sneaky trick to cope is to stand in the kitchen's industrial-sized, walk-in freezer. From plus 40° Celsius to minus 5° Celsius in an instant. The steam rises off you straight away. Another, I'm told, is to put ice cubes down your bra to cool "the girls" down— like a polar dip in a nearly frozen lake, it stings but is invigorating. Lads, it can feel like you need a spatula just to unstick "the boys" from your leg.

Naturally, it takes one to two weeks for the necessary part to be installed and thereafter reach a Goldilocks' temperature range throughout the building consistently and reliably. In the meantime, the best that can be done is to place what can only be described as industrial fans (think, diameter of almost a metre . . . with *sharp* metal blades enclosed, of course) throughout the hallways. To be clear, this doesn't actually do any cooling; rather, they simply circulate the hot, humid air (and the malodourous miasma along with it). Oh, and given that they're being run at MAX for hours on end, they're noisy, which makes communication that much more difficult. You have to remember a high proportion of residents have difficulty hearing to begin with (plus English isn't the first language of many workers). All in all, a perfect storm has been created, whereby everyone feels disgusting, and no one can understand a word that's being said to them. Spiffy.

> **NOTE**: A PSW was once suspended for "yelling at a resident." Turns out fans were running . . . and the resident was deaf, anyway. Interesting managerial approach.

Perhaps out of a sense of trying to cope through humour or out of a mild state of delirium brought about by dehydration (although most likely a combination of the two), a nurse remarked, *"When I'm schweaty, I drink Schwepps [ginger ale]."*

Staff laughed. Like the elementary school class clown, this was the very type of positive reinforcement to make a stupid play on words catchy. Schubsequently, every noun that could have the "sch" prefix added, underwent this instantaneous alteration in local dialect—'twas the first Wrinkly Ranchism.

"My name is Schynthia."

"Did you get Eleanor's schooter battery charged?"

"Did Dick get his schuppository on nights?"

All fun and games for the staff who needed a chuckle—until the resident who had been sitting at the nursing station bellowed: *I need my schhhh-weater; I'm cold.*

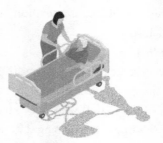

Chapter 10
HOUSEKEEPING

"Knock! Knock! Housekeep! Keepers of the house!"

This is often one of the first things residents hear in the morning (unless they haven't yet put their hearing aids in). Still, always a friendly face and, by-and-large, warmly received.

First off, it's important to acknowledge the contribution that this small team of individuals make to the global functioning of the home itself. Often, housekeeping (otherwise known in stilted language as "environmental services") hold the unenviable position of being the most-important-yet-least-recognized group in the organization. And often it's worse than that, because for whatever reason, they are perceived to sit at the bottom of the organizational totem pole of importance, glamour, or prestige.

Rubbish.

Maybe that's why poor management consider housekeeping to be nothing more than a pesky line item on the budget rather than a critical investment with a multiplier savings effect on clinicians' time and to personal protective equipment (PPE) supplies—never mind the enhancements to quality of life and ameliorated resident health-care outcomes.

HINT: If you ever need anything, want to find something/someone, or to know what's really going on, find the nearest janitor (used interchangeably with 'housekeeper' and 'environmental service worker'). It is likely that few others will be as well informed, offer a more unbiased and unvarnished opinion, or have their finger on the pulse of the organization more accurately.

Who else talks to more different people in a day? Who has a slightly removed and unaffiliated perspective? Nobody. There you go.

We can all learn from their interesting tricks of the trade too. For example, did you know that WD-40 is an amazing stainless-steel cleaner? It also wipes off gummy sticker residue better than most other products. Likewise, when mopping a floor, always keep your back straight (it's a "major danger" not to), hold your arms out and whisk the mop with your wrists; "… *it's all in the angle of the dangle*". Now you know.

Of course, there is the nitty gritty of cleaning up unmentionable spills, stripping and waxing floors (or, riding those nifty floor-cleaning Zambonis!), emptying waste and recycling receptacles, and ensuring all food preparation and dining areas are spotless. However, the most vital contribution of housekeeping is the vigilance and mindfulness applied towards perfecting their trade such that, in so doing, they stop the spread of communicable diseases, not to mention being a helpful pair of available hands whenever the clinical staff need one.

Preventing outbreaks in group-living settings is absolutely essential—particularly when otherwise vulnerable populations are at risk of being exposed. Wiping down 'touch points' (i.e., high-traffic and frequently touched surfaces) plays an integral part in stopping the spread of infections. Preventing and curtailing outbreaks have huge clinical, financial, and morale-boosting implications (besides, making sure floors are not sticky and applying a liberal amount of air freshener go a long way to making the work environment far more pleasant . . . or at least tolerable).

And nobody has a greater proportional share in these outcomes than housekeeping.

It isn't commonly understood that there are different levels of cleaning; each needs to be applied appropriately given the circumstances. During outbreaks especially, the environmental services' staff understand when simply to clean versus the need to sanitize or sterilize. To prevent the spread and hasten the end of an outbreak, enhanced measures are applied skillfully by this team. For example, such measures highlight the requirement to use the right product, in the right concentration, and for the right duration of contact time on the surface in question (the most common mistake is to wipe the cleaning product up off the dirty surface too quickly for it to be completely sterilized). Remaining cognizant to avoid cross-contamination by cleaning in the correct order (wiping from high to low and from clean to dirty) is essential (and not easy) to put into practice.

All very skillful—and vitally important—stuff.

Which makes the expectations on this small group (say, five or six people for a 50,000-square foot home) all the more bewildering. How can any one person be expected to clean (or sanitize) 5,000 to 10,000 square feet? Often by hand. In only seven hours. That's a systems' problem that ought not be borne by a such small team.

When a nurse once asked a housekeeper what the highlight of their day was, assuming it to be getting to ride the Zamboni around, the downtrodden housekeeper responded: "No, leaving." So, if you drop something or if they've missed a spot—clean it up yourself. This isn't an all-inclusive country club.

Next time you're around, please stop and thank your local housekeeper. Chances are they'll take a moment to respond, first needing to get over the shock of being complimented. They aren't used to it – and that should change.

Remember the adage: *Housekeeping! We aim to please. You, aim too, please.*

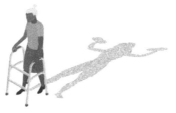

Chapter 11
RECREATION ("REC") STAFF

In any health-care-related setting, it's no surprise to find doctors, nurse practitioners, registered nurses, registered practical nurses, personal support workers, registered dietitians, physiotherapists, and so on—every denomination of clinical staff you might shake a stick at, but it doesn't stop there. You might not have considered that in long-term care, you will find a team of recreation or "life enrichment" staff.

The rec staff are a much beloved team whose sole purpose is to enhance each resident's quality of life (it's no wonder that the residents tend to prefer their company to any nurse's . . . even though they provide the warm blankets and narcotics). Families will find out quickly which member(s) of the rec staff their mother/father likes most. There are always favourites, and that's a good thing because trusting relationships always help with the speed of effective communication on important matters (mood, health status, etc.). In this regard, their perspective and observations are especially important considerations for the clinical staff; it pays to know your audience well, with respect to early detection (aka "Spidey sense") of when something isn't quite right with a resident.

The rec staff single-handedly organize and execute all games, special events (who doesn't love the Salvation Army brass band's live performances?), guest appearances (*"Elvis is IN THE BUILDING!"*), and virtual visits with outside family and friends. Word games (complete with themes), card games, colouring, pumpkin carving, putting up markets for people to go "shopping," hosting fancy-schmancy soirees (complete with doing up the ladies' nail polish, always a much-appreciated favourite!), bingo, discussing current events in the paper—you name it, they do it.

I suppose you can't become too upset when residents start to think they're on a Hawaiian love booze cruise after the rec staff have been showing episodes of *The Love Boat*. On repeat. For hours. With the volume on FULL.

As a familiar extra pair of hands, they'll help with resident transportation (i.e., wheeling people around) and feeding. Knowing residents as intimately as they do, rec staff often have a very personal anecdote to share with the group at an honour guard ceremony when a resident is leaving the building for the last time with the funeral home staff.

Rec staff will decorate for all seasonal events (one of the only ways residents know what month it is—besides, it's nice that all the beige walls are broken up with a splash of colour), facilitate religious services, celebrate every resident's birthday (with helium balloons!), and give gifts to each resident over the holiday season. We're talking an industrial operation that pays individual attention and attempts to make a personal touch for everyone—leaving nobody excluded (and they don't take offence when someone declines and is especially grumpy any particular day; tomorrow is a new day, after all). It's quite the operation.

And who doesn't love an outdoor BBQ?! (Even if they end up pureeing your hotdog.)

With the help of families, they will upload a resident's favourite music to iPods and let them rock out with headphones (in their wheelchair or with their walker)—which, by the way, is far more effective at elevating or calming someone's mood than any pharmaceutical. Just ask any staff.

Rec staff will also organize group fitness activities. It's amazing to see how much Zumba and basic band and body weight-based exercises not only elevate group mood but boost appetite, balance, basic strength, and flexibility (so important in preventing critical outcomes from falls).

And we don't even have to mention how popular animal visits are, even when the therapy dog shits in the hallway.

No wonder they're everyone's favourite. They enrich lives.

In an environment where time loses meaning (*"What day is it again? Ah, who cares? They're all the same anyway."*), life can be reduced simply to waiting for the next event (usually the next meal . . . or bath . . . or being helped to the toilet). When rec staff are around, that event—that welcome distraction, however brief—can take them away to a different place or back in time.

Beautiful legs . . . B11. *Bingo!*

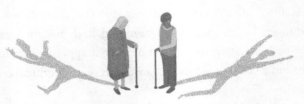

Chapter 12
LAUNDRY

Often an overlooked service—working like stink, literally and figuratively, in the background—is the industrial-scale, on-site laundry department's operation. How else might you be able to provide fresh towels, bed linens, and clothes for over 150 people? Every day. Especially when most go through more than one outfit (for various reasons . . .) on a daily basis.

Working most closely with the environmental/housekeeping department (interestingly, most staff are cross-trained between the two; you can never have too many back-ups—cross pollination is essential in maintaining uninterrupted service, after all), this small, dedicated, and hard-working group lies in the most tucked-away rooms on the premises. In the proverbial bowels of the organization is where the magic happens (i.e., removing the contents of people's bowels from linens and clothes).

It's quite a fascinating operation to witness: multiple drum-sized washers and an equal number (of equally large) dryers going every day of the week (certainly wouldn't want to pay that hydro bill). The electric motors on these machines must be able to propel a vehicle (when they're spinning at full chat, you might be forgiven for thinking they're about to take off), and the dryers' power to throw off serious heat must rival some toaster ovens' ability to burn bread. (Never tried putting in any slices of multigrain to find out, though.)

Not to mention the sorting—and not just the whites (which, by the way, arrive at laundry looking anything but . . .) from the rest of the colours, but keeping each resident's clothes (within their correct unit) organized and ready for return delivery. It's as if each resident has their own postal code.

Free pick-up and delivery (and put away in your closet and drawers!), mostly error-free. Not too shabby.

NOTE: Whenever a resident is admitted or whenever they are provided with a new item of clothing, the first thing that happens is that it is labelled. Failure to do this will, in all likelihood, result in it never being seen again. So, if you're dropping off some new socks, bra, or trousers, don't forget to ask to have them labelled. That's job *numero uno*. And this is usually done by the laundry staff.

Special shout out of appreciation to those handling the "special" loads marked "biohazard," which must be disinfected *and* sterilized (i.e., clothing not just spoiled by any regular unmentionable spills/accidents but also by any excrement of someone on cytotoxic, anti-cancer drugs). Enough said.

Another unwritten yet invaluable service provided by the mindful laundry staff is their constant vigilance for missing items. As silly as it sounds, it's incredible what ends up getting laundered: hearings aids, dentures, TV remotes, unmarked dildos—you name it. Yet, provided they still work upon return, they at least look brand new. The dentures especially always sparkle after a good bleaching, as if the resident just had their teeth whitened.

But don't worry, your "delicates" and secrets are safe—they never air people's dirty laundry.

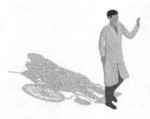

Chapter 13
WORKING WITH FOREIGN-TRAINED PROFESSIONALS

We live and work in a multicultural society. Nowhere is that more evident than in health care. Naturally, the English language is not native to everyone; consequently, challenges to effective communication can result.

To be perfectly clear, I enjoy working with everyone and the sense of comradery that stems from collaborating with friendly, professional and collegial teammates who place no bias on 'class' of employee. We need everyone and everyone needs us. In fact, I once had a coach who preached the following sage advice (admittedly over my head at the time): *"Holy Snappers! Nobody is above the teeeeeeam, big guy!"*

Truer words have never been spoken.

I find that those trained overseas to be especially polite and (*very*) well educated (don't be surprised if the person sweeping the floor or bathing your resident was a physician, pharmacist or PhD in their country of origin)—so this chapter is in no way an indictment of ability. In fact, those born overseas often demonstrate a tireless work ethic (that those born here ought to emulate), quiet perseverance, and selfless dedication to the job, the residents, and their team. That said, amusing misunderstandings do occur and a representative sample of mishaps, miscommunications, and misadventures follow.

Sometimes, the resulting snafus are innocuous . . . and make you chuckle. For example, when asking for a paper clip, the person was given (*enthusiastically* to be so helpful and eager to please) a paper cup. Trying to explain the difference took a while.

Or once, when walking the staff member through using a computer program, they apologized, stating that they were not that *"tech swabby."*

Or realizing that the new temporary worker's name was indeed *Friendli.* . . and that they were really nice, too. Deliciously funny irony (and a helpful mnemonic for their name).

Or asking if the staff member would like something to eat or drink (as part of the communal coffee order) only for them to decline, stating that they have their own *"Baileys"* (at work?!); upon clarification, they were eating berries.

One holiday, after getting into the Christmas spirit (given all the music playing, blaring rather), one jolly and well-meaning staff member started skipping down the hall singing, *"Horny! Horny! Horny!"* After taking the staff member aside, another explained (with a straight face) that "horny," in English, means a state of arousal, typically when describing a man but applies equally to a woman, and suggested that, perhaps, they had meant to sing, *"Holly! Holly! Holly!"* They agreed.

Or when a native English speaker self-indulged and capitalized on the opportunity to remark, *"No way, José!"* when they spoke with incredulity to a staff by that very name . . . and they didn't understand why it was funny.

Sometimes, it is just plain confusing.

Imagine trying to take shift report (a summary, hand-over conversation to transfer responsibility from the exiting nurse to the nurse coming on duty) and discussing individual residents with someone who either confuses and/or interchanges personal pronouns randomly (i.e., they will use 'she' and 'he' when discussing the same resident). For example: *"Margaret hit his head when she fell next to Paul's walker. He's okay, and she bruised his elbow."*

"So, is Paul okay or Margaret? Or both? Whose elbow is bruised?"

See the difficulty here?

Another example from a hand-off report: when describing the location of a wound, they stated it was on the left foot, middle finger. Huh?!

And it's not just the staff. From a resident perspective, imagine being in your nineties, being hard of hearing, and trying to make sense of what someone wearing a mask is trying to say when English isn't their first language (i.e., thick accent) and all while the TV is blaring in the background so loudly it sounds like a rock concert.

One day, a relatively new staff member misinterpreted a resident's name, and schubsequently, a male resident found bras in his wardrobe. He tried to put them on as underwear and remarked: *"Nice padding."*

Sometimes, it stops and makes you wonder.

For example, after a foreign, vegan staff member continuously extolled their virtuous lifestyle and gastronomic choices, they couldn't be found because they were on their second smoke break of the morning.

Given that the vast majority of workers were foreign-born, it struck a nurse one day that perhaps the next time management decides to play the national anthem, it might be more fitting to play the Filipino, Indian, or Mexican one.

Sometimes, differences result in conflict.

The ugly side and equally incredulous: one day, a nurse walked into a room to find two foreign-born staff squabbling, each accusing the other of having bad English—true story! Try getting to the bottom of that international diplomatic mess. Since when does the nurse need to be an ambassador of foreign relations?

Just call me Switzerland.

Another time, a nurse had to stand up for the care team on duty when the foreign-born son of a palliative resident (whom we hadn't seen in the ten plus years their parent had been a resident . . . just wanted to point that out) was all in everyone's face and condescending specifically (and ironically) to the foreign-born staff (albeit of a different nationality). All because he believed 'Dr. Google' over the care team's advice. Going out of his way to besmirch them personally was a particularly classless touch. Uncouth, unnecessary, and unacceptable.

Loser.

Maybe it's just best to listen to more Christmas music. The horny kind.

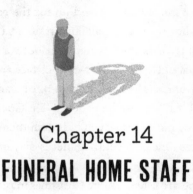

Chapter 14
FUNERAL HOME STAFF

The denizens of any long-term care home.

Funeral home staff are a lovely, convivial sort, but they are also the kind who present as slightly too enthusiastic about their job (we all know the type) and are typically, and rather ironically, old enough to be the next in line to lay on the gurney. Makes you question what's going on (have they really seen *that many* dead bodies that they've lost all sense of the moment's gravitas?). Still, it's always nice to see a friendly smiling face, I suppose.

Whenever a resident passes away "at home" within the facility and after any local family/friends have had ample opportunity to say their final goodbyes, some rudimentary documentation needs to be completed because, as anyone working in health care will tell you, you can never have too much documentation (the CYA rule never ceases to apply—even in death).

At this time, you may be surprised to learn that a significant portion of families have not yet made after-death arrangements—like, they have *no* plan in place (did they think their parents were going to live forever?!). Naturally, they look to the nursing staff for direction (as if it were part of the full concierge, country-club service) and, schubsequently, are coached through the process. Nurses know that, although they didn't receive any such official training, they may have to act as social workers and care for an entire family, not just for the resident.

> **HINT:** If you don't yet have a will, or if it needs to be updated, *do it now*. Make sure you talk about and share your wishes with those who will be responsible for your future care and estate. Seek the auspicious moment, have the awkward, adult conversation and be prepared – don't be a day late and dollar short on this one. Getting push-back? Tell them to stop, listen and to focus on the present reality, no matter how much they may wish to avoid the topic. If you don't, on your head be it.

Before a body is ready to be taken by the funeral home personnel, the nursing staff will ensure that the resident has been changed and washed as necessary (many people soil themselves after death . . . once everything relaxes) and any "tubes" have been removed (e.g., IVs, urinary catheters, or palliative medication ports, often known as "butterflies"). A clean outfit will be put on, as per the family's preference. All components of an impressively dignified level of care.

Transferring the body from the bed to the folding wheeled gurney (it's got to fit back into the hearse, after all) is always a . . . unique process. Depending on the room's dimensions and layout and the clutter/hoarding within it, it can be a challenge to sidle the gurney up to the bed.

With any transfer where you're essentially sliding a body from the bed to a stretcher or gurney, how easy or difficult it is will depend entirely on the individual's size, weight, and mobility; being a dead weight (literally) or as stiff as Peter North doesn't necessarily make it easier. Normally, the body is then placed in a zip-up body bag and buckled in (why *two* seat belts are necessary, I don't know), so it doesn't fly off the gurney in travel (the laws of physics still apply, even in death).

It's the one-off situations that are especially memorable, if a bit sketchy. Like the time the gurney could barely fit into the room because the resident had been a hoarder, so it was just easier to pick the dead body up off the bed (one at the head, one at the feet) and heave them onto the gurney (at which point, the gurney almost toppled over, and the body nearly rolled off)—*glad the door was closed for that one.*

Or the time the body had been left sitting upright in bed a little too long after death . . . and had since stiffened in a V-shaped position. Good old *rigor mortis.* Then we really did need the second seat belt to flatten them out, and even then, the body bag looked like a giant strained erection.

Or the time a bariatric (a very heavy person, typically in excess of 400 pounds) resident's body couldn't fit into the body bag (let alone get buckled in), which was rather awkward, to say the least. With a sheet drawn over them, they looked like a muffin on wheels (*ironic, no?*) and made the strained wheels squeak and grind all the way to the hearse. And all you can do is pray the frame doesn't buckle. Dodgy at best.

And speaking of hearses, you might be surprised to know that the vehicle usually used to pick up the bodies from the home is nothing more than a slightly modified, unmarked minivan (the type that's raised with no back windows). So, the next time you pass such a vehicle, you may want to think twice about the fact that there might be a dead body in the back (and sometimes, two if it's been a "busy" day).

In one particularly memorable instance, the family remarked that their loved one always wanted a ride in a Benz – and finally got it – as the resident's body was loaded into the back of the black diesel Mercedes Sprinter van. I could barely contain my laughter until one of them they said: "Drive safely!" at which point, I burst out. (Just like the Barenaked ladies sing: "I'm the type of guy who laughs at a funeral." *Sorry, can't help it.*)

Wonder what they might say to the police if they were every pulled over . . . for not coming to a "dead" stop at an intersection. That might take some explaining.

Tight spaces, Peter North, a squeaky muffin on wheels, and riding off in a Benz—what a way to go out!

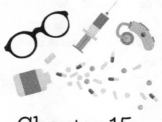

Chapter 15
INS AND OUTS

"How much did you eat today? What proportion of your meals did you eat? Snacks? How many glasses did you drink (or were thickened and spoon-fed to you)? Are you regular? Enjoy a particularly thorough evacuation of your bowels this morning? No? Been a couple of days, has it?"

How would you like being asked all this . . . *every* day? Well, get used to it.

In LTC, it's common practice (for a variety of reasons) to take each resident's weight on a monthly basis. High-tech lifts (the type that are used to move a resident from a bed to a chair, or from a chair to a toilet, for example) may have a built-in weight scale. Depending on if weight gain is observed, schubsequent changes to that resident's diet (and/or medications) may follow.

Except, know that you can't always make one change in isolation without experiencing a cascade of unintended side effects.

NOTE: In terms of quality of life, the sense of taste usually sees the least amount of deterioration as we age (chocolate cake will always taste good, even if you can't see it or hear the people asking if you want any).

As much as staff attempt to document intake accurately, miscalculations occur easily if residents snack independently (more often, brought in for them by family/friends) . . . or eat others' food. Or give theirs away. Or throw it up. Or throw it across the room (with or without their dentures).

What you may not expect is the amount of attention paid to how much a resident voids (pees) or how frequently they empty their bowels (shits). Euphemistically, this is often called "having a bowel movement" (or, shortened to 'BM'). In fact, there's a charming pictorial diagram called the Bristol Stool Chart (hand on heart, this is a real thing—*Google it right now*) that describes the types of excrement as a quick reference for staff wanting to document accurately (think, *"firm sausage-shaped with lines"* to *"fluffy cloud"* to *"pure liquid"*).

And here you thought that poop was a taboo subject and a blight on the physical or conversational landscape. Quite the opposite.

NOTE: Interestingly, there isn't a clear category for the enormous turd that emerges after five days without any movement: where the heavens open and the resident gives birth to what can only be described as a heap in the shape of a football. And about the same size (must have hurt coming out). *Touchdown!* But hey, *the bigger the pile, the bigger the smile.* Only then to clog the toilet—whereupon the nearest member of housekeeping or maintenance has to go get "the stick" to break it up and poke it down. Seriously.

Rather innocently, one nurse remarked that after disimpacting a resident (after Day 5 without a movement), they wished that the huge heap of turds was instead *"a mountain of golden nuggets."*

Cute.

Residents with a catheter have their "output" measured and documented and then compared to how much they had to drink (men, if you don't know what a catheter is, think of it as a tube that's inserted up your old chap . . . right up until it gets into your bladder. It's as uncomfortable as it sounds and will make you shrivel till it's a "button on a fur coat"—*how vexatious!*). Measuring accurately gets tougher when catheters get pulled out (with the balloon still inflated! Can you imagine how much that must hurt?!) or if urine bypasses the catheter (which happens when there isn't a snug fit and piss comes out the sides).

Naturally, all such attention is paid because good care ensures that people balance being well nourished and hydrated with the medical needs of ensuring any unhealthy (and potentially dangerous) retention is avoided and treated promptly.

Couple of challenges with this seemingly simple goal: First, many residents are relatively sedentary, spending most of their days either lying in bed or sitting in a chair. Second, frequent and regular consumption of narcotic pain killers are not uncommon, which are known to have the unfortunate side effect of slowing down the body's ability to clear stool (poop). The cumulative effect of these realities is that people often don't have a BM every day, despite straining to do so (fondly referred to as *"trying to shit through the eye of a needle"*). Some go days despite increasingly invasive interventions to get "things moving." When was the last time you went two days without a poop? Three? Five?! How uncomfortable would you be?

Did you hear about the constipated mathematician? They worked it out with a pencil.

But . . . sometimes residents manage to toilet themselves and then either forget or don't tell the staff. Or go in another's washroom (so their "deposit" is attributed to someone else). Or, simply lean against the door to their room and piss into the hallway. Or into the nearest garbage can. Or into the plant pots (just look for the dead ones). Predictably, this results in staff thinking one thing but the reality being very different. On comes the bowel regimen until definitive results are obtained: oral stool softeners, suppositories . . . and enemas.

As an aside, a high proportion of resident falls are attributable to them attempting to get to the washroom independently (it's always a good idea to remind an older adult to ring the bell any time they need assistance). This is why there ought to be a call bell placed within easy reach of their bed and chair; remember always: "*Call, don't fall!*"

Residents with poor memories will forget that they've eaten before having left the dining room; they will forget that they've been toileted immediately after being sat back in their chairs. This often results in them struggling to get back up—only for the staff to reassure them and ask that they remain seated (for their own safety). Up and down like a toilet seat they go for what seems to take forever.

A personal favourite occurs when a resident finally goes (after umpteen doses of stool softeners) only then to have, predictably, a LARGE loooose movement. *Sweet relief!* BUT as loose stool may be interpreted as a sign of an infectious outbreak, the resident is then placed into isolation for twenty-four to seventy-two hours. So, now you're caught in a cycle of either being bunged up . . . or in lockdown. All because your shit ain't right.

Damned if you doo-doo. Damned if you don't.

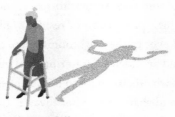

Chapter 16
SAGGY STUFF

We all will experience the physical ravages of time on a more or less equal basis. As the title suggests, this might not be the most uplifting chapter—but one worth working through because its universality is omnipresent.

This is why residents feel absolute equanimity farting out loud in the dining room as they might more privately elsewhere (hey, at least you know they're still breathing). They know that Dickie at the table over by the window will no doubt be doing the same at any moment (heck, time it right and you might get away with it—blame all the trumpeting on him; that's what the staff do, anyway). Sometimes, people "gamble and win" (i.e., don't shit their pants when they pass gas), and sometimes, they "gamble and lose." You can usually tell by the fart's crescendo of rectal velocity to make an educated guess as to the eventual outcome. That and the squishy shifting in the seat afterwards.

Take Eunice, who always gets her best sleep in the dining room at breakfast after being up all night; her top dentures clinging on for dear life (after dropping off the upper-level gums and almost flying out with every exhalation), that is, until she snores so loudly, she wakes herself up. Her tablemates don't bat an eye and make sure she's got the food she prefers waiting for her when she does—it is a community, after all.

It's remarkably humbling to watch people fall to bits (i.e., lose much physical functionality, unless of course they're an amputee and can't get their leg on) but soldier on nonetheless without ego, embarrassment, or shame because it just isn't as important as eating that slice of bacon or chocolate cake. Might be their last.

"I'm old, not dead!" Often comes to mind.

In a way, it puts our normal fastidious attention to preening and obsessive masking of all bodily functions to shame.

Here's a couple more-common-than-you-might-believe, gender-based examples (for parity, of course):

- **Men:** Your testicles drop, sometimes to alarmingly low levels (think, almost-to-your-knees). Maybe it just looks exaggerated next to how your penis has shrivelled up, which makes one wonder why this happens (do your testicles lose the ability to self-regulate their optimum operating temperature or does that skin lose THAT much elasticity?!). This has actual care implications; it isn't uncommon for a man's testicles to end up resting on the top of the heap of their Day 5 bowel movement (or, less often, in the toilet's cold water). Therefore, it's best to make sure they get wiped off separately and flung upwards when placed in a brief (respectful euphemism for adult diaper)—sitting on them is incredibly uncomfortable.

- **Women:** Your breasts sag. Staff have to watch they don't get tucked into the belt of your pants while you're sitting in a wheelchair. And that the skin under the fold doesn't get a heat rash from not being dried properly.

As age-old the joke goes: if you don't get some support for the girls, people will think they're nuts!

... but enough of the low hanging fruit.

As older adults' skin loses its elasticity and wrinkles abound, it's actually a great metaphor – their skin isn't 'loose', it's just a 'relaxed fit'. And maybe that's how we should approach the aging process.

Eat dessert first. As if it's your last. Never mind any malodourous Bronx cheers from those around you. It's better that they're there, even if they blame you for the smell.

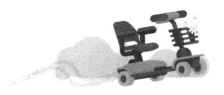

Chapter 17
WATCH OUT!

(NOT EVERYTHING MOVES SLOWLY AROUND HERE)

A long-term care hallway isn't the type of setting one might suspect as being particularly dangerous . . . but you'd be wrong. Speed demons lurk in your midst. Or, more likely, people just half asleep or drugged up (or both) at the wheel. You'd be surprised at how quickly battery-operated electronic scooters and wheelchairs can go—and the havoc they can cause.

All you're missing are some sweet jumps, and you'd have Evel Knievel (albeit with thick glasses and wearing a brief) zinging around with one hand on the wheel and the other waving their cane with an air of commanding imperiousness. The way some do, you wonder if they're trying their best Evel impersonation (some oversteer and resulting power slides on wet linoleum floor do point to some modest underlying skill) . . . or reliving their youth. Can't blame them, really.

It's interesting to watch how driving has permeated our culture so entirely. Residents hold on to their driving "privileges" like Charlton to his rifle—to the bitter end. Ultimately, residents will have their motors disengaged after one too many ramrod "bumper car" accidents. Just ask the local maintenance crew how many times they've had to repatch the drywall (in entire sections). All scooters can reverse, but few residents do. And it only causes problems when they do (ever seen a true eighteen-point turn?!).

Of course, most drive like Miss Daisy . . . because they are. However, there is nothing quite as funny as seeing them mistake the throttle knob for something else and turn up their dinged-up, paint-chipped, flower-clad, basket-toting rocket ships from turtle to full rabbit; the moment they grip the hand-throttle, their heads snap back in shock. Most release the throttle at the same time as they release their bowels—both as natural reflexes of pure surprise: "*Gad zukes!*"

Others grow impatient of those who block the halls and do not have electronic mobility. The pitch of the horns found on these modest means of conveyance belie an undertone of pure aggression. 'scooter spite' is the geriatric equivalent of 'road rage'. Nothing quite so remarkable as someone trying to *rush* to the dining room for breakfast even though they're still an hour early (but since they've been up since 4:30 a.m., you can understand their desire to get on with the day). Unfortunately, they're held up by someone who's since fallen asleep in their own wheelchair (because they've been up all night) in the middle of the hallway. No amount of standing on the horn will either wake them or make them move faster. In contrast, others whose hearing aids (with new batteries!) are in place are frightened half to death by the shock of a horn . . . and pee their pants at the slightest *beep! beep!*

But the antics don't stop there. Oh no.

After suffering one too many near misses from being run over, good old Ethel snuck out of her room after bedtime (i.e., wheeled herself three doors down) to unplug Paul's scooter's battery charger. A premeditated surgical strike if ever there was one. When Paul woke up the next morning, the scooter hadn't charged and its battery was flat. He was dead in the water. Vigilante justice had been served.

Even-steven.

But it's not just the residents. Staff are just as guilty of banging up the walls with carts (large metal laundry carts are the biggest offenders). And it's not just the halls that take a beating: While kneeling to attend to a resident, I was hit right in the middle of the forehead with a lift that was wheeled in (lowered all the way) to raise the resident from where they had fallen on the floor. Thankfully, I didn't soil myself . . . and everyone had a good laugh at my expense. Even the resident.

Watch out!

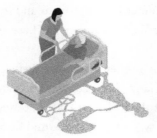

Chapter 18
BATH TIME, FUN TIME!

One activity of daily living (ADL) that is among the first to cause a significant challenge as people age at home concerns the delicate subject of hygiene. In particular, bathing is especially difficult and rife with slip/fall risks for a variety of reasons: often people fall and break a hip, and so begins the downward spiral of their overall independence and health prognosis (i.e., it's a common catalyst for people ending up requiring long-term care).

As a result, one of the greatest pleasures for those newly admitted to a LTC home is that they get to enjoy a nice hot bath in a safe environment, if only a couple of times per week (unless of course they have a huge "accident" and then it's time for a total tune-up). Logistically speaking, ensuring every resident stays up to date on their bathing schedule, given the myriad challenges faced by the staff daily, isn't easy. Yet, somehow, the front-line caregivers—the PSWs—the real miracle workers (let's be honest), make it work.

Typically, there are only one or two tubs per unit, as they are part of complex "tub rooms" (with ceiling lifts, waterproof chair lifts, and motorized tubs that can raise and lower). It's a pretty neat set-up, in actual fact.

Naturally, as with most aspects of living/working in LTC, scarcely believable events occur organically, at which you can't help but just laugh.

For example, albeit based upon potty humour, whenever a resident is truly relaxed in the warm water, it isn't uncommon for them to pass wind (perhaps the soothing warmth acting as the final ingredient to get things moving from being bunged up?). What's particularly funny is when a frail, petite, older woman surprises herself when the perfect ass-cheek-to-tub-surface ratio results in the loudest resonating fart that can be heard through closed doors, halfway down the hall. Brrrrrrpp! ("*What the hell was that?!*")

Another example: Whenever a particular gentleman had his bath day, fortunately for him, his doting wife would come into the home to relieve him with her loving touch. That's dedication and commitment if I've ever seen it (and likely better than any narcotic . . . or sleep aid). Again, these people are old, not dead. In the same vein, a *soapy helicopter* is always good for a laugh.

A third example highlights the "help" some family members offer staff. After assisting staff to bathe their foreign-born (but English-speaking . . . when they wanted to) parent, the adult child of the resident insisted that their parent had had a bowel movement while in the tub. This was significant because it negated the need for further intervention to bring on a bowel movement—you would think, a good thing. However, when the staff couldn't confirm there was any "*chi-chi kaa-kaa*" lurking "under the bubbles," it was cause for consternation. It wasn't like the tub was clogged and couldn't drain, and the staff certainly didn't . . . poke the "water" down the hole.

Clean as a whistle, feeling empty and relieved—bath time, fun time!

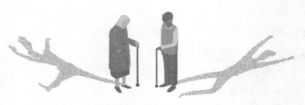

Chapter 19
LET'S TALK ABOUT SEX, BABY!

Who said that having no teeth was a bad thing? Sometimes having removable dentures has an upside....

Keen observers will by now recognize the recurrent and main thrust of this book's thesis: older adults are just that . . . adults. They are alive, not dead. And as much as parts of people stop working as they get older, hormonal drives can remain resolutely determined (as evidenced by some residents acting out their fantasies of being handsome Chad Thundercock Lotharios... in the buff). This may come as a surprise (no pun intended), but lust and love usually find a way—a cliché but true.

The ethereal beauty of sex isn't just a pursuit of the young. Open your mind to this reality as many a dalliance as been known to occur.

From the most innocent and spontaneous holding of hands to the most intimate of acts, the entire range of otherwise normal adult sexual behaviour may go on in LTC (and not always with the person's partner; sometimes husband and wife couples, both admitted, don't even live in the same unit, let alone the same room. In contrast, others may remain entirely inseparable). Residents who are single (as a good proportion are, in actual fact) often enjoy the company of others now that it's once again easy to meet people.

That prospect might put some lead in the old pencil.

Perhaps it's the realization that whatever consequences might have been feared in the past are now viewed in a new light, or maybe it's a result of boredom, loneliness, or dementia, but some residents can become rather (and surprisingly) uninhibited—sometimes publicly (i.e., kissing every person passionately as they wander down the hall). For example, residents wandering luridly semi or fully nude down the hallways (and into others' rooms . . . or closets or beds) is not uncommon (and not necessarily off-putting to the others, either—it's all perspective, after all). Regardless, being comfortable is number one, so it's not uncommon to see people adjust themselves, scratch their asses, or pick their noses publicly. *Unnnnnnbelievable.*

Similarly, having multiple "relationships" simultaneously is not unheard of (is it cheating if both parties suffer from dementia?!). Do you permit two seemingly happy residents from spending time together if they are both unable to provide consent due to their advanced dementia?

Sexually transmitted infections are also considerations in pharmacological treatment. Lifelong infections sometimes manifest as immune systems wane (*"When good old Henry returned after the War, he brought something else home with him. . . ."*).

Rather awkwardly for staff, some especially gregarious residents may form unsolicited attachments. Naturally, these can range from engaging in good-natured, mild, flirtatious banter marked by innocent frivolity (*"You're so cute!"*) to making salacious remarks (*"When busty Lisa rushes down the hall, it's like a couple of bear cubs are fighting under a blanket"*) and can escalate to groping staff inappropriately. Fair or otherwise, this makes for solid ethical debate on issues of ability to provide (implied?) consent, mental competence, and guilt versus responsibility for inappropriate and conniving behaviours.

As a front-line clinician, if you take the approach that sexual exploits and their consequences are just as normal (and predictable) as other bodily functions, it will come as no surprise that some people will masturbate (aka 'feed the geese' or 'flick your bean') even if that means walking in to a resident's room as they watch porn . . . often with the volume turned up so loud that it can be heard all the way down the hall (*is this a care facility or a brothel?!*). Sometimes with the (mis)use of objects—a not uncommon example highlights the many alternative uses of electric toothbrushes; it's amazing how fast those batteries will go flat with constant and heavy use. (*What came first, the yeast infection or all the masturbation? What's really "itchy" down there?!*)

In one unforgettable incident, a new resident's dildo was accidentally knocked off their bedside table and, upon hitting the floor, turned itself on, only to vibrate and gyrate *vigorously*. After the initial shock and moment of silent embarrassment of the staff, everyone couldn't help but bust out in laughter . . . and this went on until, after several rather delicate attempts to pick it up had failed, someone bellowed: *"Just grab it by the shaft!"* Everyone was in stitches. Literally dead.

> **NOTE:** You might be surprised to learn that there could be nearly as many dildos in your local LTC home as there are in the nearest sex shop.

At times, residents are totally up-front regarding matters of their libido: *"Are all these pills good for my sex life?"* Wasn't expecting that . . . and not sure how to respond either (truthfully, anyway).

Some things you simply can't un-see. Heck, maybe St. Anthony of Padua (patron Saint of the elderly) is looking out for geriatric "happiness."

For example, when residents request to be prescribed Viagra, the nursing staff can't help but advocate on their behalf (there's a markedly reduced fall risk now that they won't roll out of bed—or so the joke goes). When asked afterwards, one priapic gentleman, with a twinkle in his eyes, stated quite matter-of-factly: *"Well, I got the erection all right but could have done without the last half hour."*

Up like a rocket. Down like a feather. I guess you really can have too much of a good thing.

The tricky part comes when you need to balance promoting resident independence and choice with safeguarding them against themselves (i.e., repeated use of the toothbrush results in tissue damage and a urinary tract infection). Usually, the schubsequently required disclosure with the resident's adult children comes unexpectedly and is understandably uncomfortable (does anything quite prepare you for that?!). Very little else turns otherwise articulate adults into such taciturn beings. Especially if the new toothbrush in question didn't even belong to their parent (and they need *another* new one).

Often, the staff approach and cope with the sexual exploits of residents with equanimity (and are not at all condescending). For example, the audible cries, moans, and grunts of those yelling out as they climax (*"Where will we find the white slime today?!"*) or the unflinching, pithy, preemptive excited self-murmuring: *"Up it goes! Up it goes!"* simply underline that you're never too old to look forward to a good orgasm, and you shouldn't be embarrassed by that either.

(Privately, these sexploits can make the staff a tad jealous that they haven't enjoyed a similarly gratifying orgasm in ages). Nobody should be nonplussed by this. No need to be reticent. Just accept it.

You have to admire the youthful comments made by residents jokingly: *"I'd shave, but my girlfriend likes me a bit scruffy. It's part of my allure. Don't tell my wife!"* [who is also a resident on the same unit . . . in the same room] To remark that he was a horse of a different colour would be an understatement.

One deadpan shocker was: *"Man alive, you have to be so pussy-licking friendly to everyone around here, eh?!"*

Another: *"There are so many single women here, I could be busier than a dog with two. . . ."*

"Richard, that's enough." What a rascal. That cagey rapscallion just smirks, winks, and gives you the thumbs up.

And to think you thought that life in LTC was always dull.

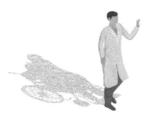

Chapter 20
HAIR IN NEW PLACES AND EAR WAX

Don't worry. This isn't going to be another awkward Grade 5 type of "birds and the bees" conversation. Nevertheless, one still worth having.

As hormone levels change, so too does hair growth. No matter, as the staff are typically very attentive, particularly towards keeping up the dignified appearance of female residents. You might be surprised to learn that "the bearded lady" isn't that far off an apt description of the facial (and arm . . . and leg . . . and everything else) hair women can grow if left unchecked.

Particularly attentive and caring workers will go out of their way to ensure faces are shaved discreetly (particularly if family are visiting). Unibrows gotta go, too. It can be an uncomfortable conversation to have with families as to why their mother/grandmother needs so many razors and shaving cream.

Men sprout rogue eyebrows or hair from their ears and nose. Thick stuff that makes a Chia Pet look strangely normal (not to mention the Wolf Man). Interestingly, there seems to be an inverse relationship between how bald a man becomes and the increased amount of hair sprouting everywhere else, all over his body.

Rather awkwardly, staff are, at times, requested to shave a resident's pubic hair . . . or not to touch it at all. Totally dependent on direction received from family.

All part of a day's work, really. Just roll with it.

Something else that tends to happen in advanced age is the increase in production of ear wax. Tons of the stuff . . . from a light honey colour and consistency to hard, dark brown (think, candle wax). Imagine how much better you'd feel being able to hear again with the removal of what could pass visually for a caramel. You're going to need a heck of a lot more than a Q-tip to get that out.

This can actually become a problem if left unchecked as it can totally clog/occlude the ear. When it does, daily oil drops will be prescribed for the better part of a week to soften the wax up before any attempt is made to remove it.

When the nurse goes in to wash it out (usually with warm water sprayed in gently), there may be other surprises to be discovered: ears clogged with cotton balls, pills, or bits of food aren't uncommon findings. It can take several cycles of oil drops and weekly rinsing to get the ear clear.

Naturally, this isn't a comfortable process for the resident but one they (and the nurse!) tend to find satisfying once complete (like the satisfaction you'd get from popping a big zit and the contents hitting the mirror). Removing a large chunk of wax is extremely satisfying—*"Ugh, SO GOOD!"*

So now you know.

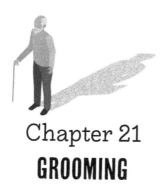

Chapter 21
GROOMING

It might seem obvious, but it's worth underlining: as you age and your faculties diminish, you rely on others to steer you right and help you with what you used to be able to do completely independently. No shame in admitting you've lost a step.

Personal grooming is a particularly obvious area that highlights the challenges on keeping up with the body's daily maintenance requirements. Despite the staff's best intensions and efforts, there is only so much personal attention that can be paid to hair, nails, teeth, strength, and flexibility. While there are sound arguments that underline why non-essential aspects of care are not a top priority in the face of other medical requirements, when one looks at the total care being offered to those who are totally dependent, it speaks to quality of life.

For example, ask any man who has had a moustache for over thirty years what's more important: pants or proper care of his handlebars? Pants lose every time (and besides, you can't see them when you're sitting down, anyway). It's all about pride of place. So, how can things go wrong with the simplest aspects of daily living and care? Well, consider that if nails are not trimmed, they grow sharp and one can quite easily hurt themselves, other residents, or staff (*don't get nailed!*) as they try to provide care. Many a skin tear and cut —on staff as much as any other resident—has happened as a result of "claws and talons."

Hazard of the job.

Oral hygiene is an area of care that is particularly challenging. Often, tooth decay will accelerate once a resident enters long-term care. If you are a family member or advocate of a resident, you are well advised to ask about what can be reasonably expected with respect to oral care (it may be something you wish to take on yourself). Oral health is absolutely key to overall health, and you really can't have one without the other.

The importance of good oral health, however, doesn't diminish if a resident has dentures; making sure they remain clean and properly fitting is key. It's also worth noting that it's best practice to label as many possessions as possible, including the denture's case. What you don't want is someone else mistaking a pair of dentures for their own. It may seem silly but isn't unheard of for people to wear someone else's dentures (yes, it's as off-putting as it sounds). When this happens, it isn't always obvious, like when a smaller size fits easily into a larger mouth; however, when someone tries to use dentures far too large for their mouth, you can't help but laugh at what then looks like the largest smile ever (even if they're having the worse day).

Dentures often go missing too. All it takes is someone removing (or sneezing . . . or spitting) them out while in bed for them to end up in the laundry. Then, it's an elaborate process of elimination to determine to whom they might belong.

The unsolicited mullet haircut has also been known to occur (when all the family requested was a trim); guess good old *Samurai Suzie* found a bowl in the kitchen and took the sides down right to the wood. . . . Despite the namesake, that most certainly does *not* result in all business up front and all party at the back (even though some mullets are so legendary that could be entered into a prize-awarding contest).

The last aspect of daily maintenance is that of physical activity with respect to the pursuit of maintaining strength (and, as a corollary, bone density), flexibility, and balance. While recreational and physical therapy staff make determined efforts to retain maximal functionality in the safest manner possible, it is never enough.

Families, one of the most useful things you can do when you visit is simply to walk with your family member for as long as they can tolerate it safely (besides, it'll help keep them regular). Don't bring them doughnuts; instead, help them brush their teeth.

Tough love, but they'll appreciate the tune-up.

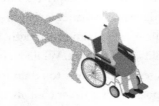

Chapter 22
TOILETING

(WARNING: THIS WILL BE MORE THAN JUST POTTY HUMOUR)

Do you poop on a schedule? Enjoying your morning ablutions so regularly that you could set a watch to them? Got yourself into a nice routine? *Sweet sphincter!* Lucky you . . . enjoy it. Others aren't so fortunate.

How would you feel if you were unable to go to the bathroom by yourself? Pretty vulnerable, I suspect. Being at the mercy of someone else/other people to help you with the whole process snuffs out any sense of independence. And dignity.

Never mind having to wear the adult version of a diaper (a 'brief' in correct geri-speak) because the team may not always be able to get to you in time. How infantilizing.

This is also complicated by several factors . . . so you can't even try to time your eating/drinking to enforce a predictive schedule, one where you could reasonably expect someone to be available to help you when you naturally feel the urge to go. Oh, spiffy.

Imagine you were given medication every day that, as a side effect, bunged you up. And once you've gotten well and truly clogged, they give you different medications to clear you out. And prunes. And maybe even a suppository for good measure (let's not even consider the frightful prospect of the next step . . . an enema).

A resident once shared that while he would rather be able to go back to having a sex life and regular, frequent orgasms, the best he could hope for now was a good bowel movement—the type of explosive detonation that leaves you feeling well and truly empty—once every three days. *Once in three days*—think about that. How would you feel having waited that long? He went on to compare the frustration of waiting and waiting (while sitting on the can) only for nothing to come of it—and then being in an almighty hurry—as not unlike the feeling of travelling and rushing/arriving/waiting/rushing in an airport.

"You're up-and-down like a toilet seat – trying to shit through the eye of a needle."

We can all identify feeling the sudden urge and needing to . . . *rush (!)*—otherwise known as the "green apple quickstep." This is to say nothing of the gambling that happens when one tries to relieve oneself of pent-up, pressurized flatulence only to have a dingleberry or two escape in the crop-dusting process—hence the need to be toileted in good time. Such "gambling and losing" results in discomforting and vexatious skid marks . . . the type that often soak through the seat of the pants for public display.

You win some. You lose some.

A portable toilet (basically a chair with a built-in, removable bucket) is called a commode. Fondly, the wider, larger-sized commode (used to accommodate more generously-proportioned or even bariatric residents) is often referred to by the staff as the "super bowl."

As you age, the onset of having to go is more immediate (things lose their elasticity, after all). So, whereas in your youth, you might have been able to sense the impending doom with considerable advanced warning, now it's . . . nothing, nothing, nothing . . . *"Oh, shit! I gotta go NOW."* Then you'll hit the call bell to ring for help and just sit there and hope . . . and pray . . . and hope someone comes before you blow because you simply can't hold it in any more.

Unless, of course, you have a catheter in place, which then follows you everywhere you go . . . and is a nice little show-and-tell piece tied around the bottom of your leg/ankle. Fashion statement aside, the benefits of no longer being incontinent of urine are offset by the schubsequently heightened risks of getting (recurrent) urinary tract infections (UTIs; which can result in increased confusion and a cascade of other issues), among other bugs. Keeping a catheter clean isn't easy either.

The staff are empathetic. They're trying their level best to get to everyone in time; if they could, they would. These are kind-hearted people. But until mankind devises a way to be in two places at once, there is little hope.

So, let's say there's a well-oiled, fully staffed care team on today. And today's the day for your big movement. You think the coffee and prunes at breakfast did the trick, as well as the tiny cup of laxative oil you asked for to be mixed in your orange juice . . . and the "magic bullet" (aka suppository) they woke you at 5:30 a.m. to "slide it up there." A couple hours later, you feel like a hand grenade and they just pulled out the pin; the clock is ticking and there's simply no going back or stopping the inevitable. Fortunately, the PSWs have managed to get you lifted (with a mechanical lift) from your wheelchair to the toilet in time, and you strain to do your business (because it's such a big, hard turd, and it's putting up a fight… despite the pressure) when suddenly you feel light-headed.

The care team comes in moments later to check in on you, and you've passed out. Your blood pressure is "sixty/dead;" you have suffered what's called a vasovagal episode (basically, your blood pressure drops temporarily and you faint). Good news is that the light-headedness passes, and you're feeling much better for having emptied your bowels. It's a good thing the team left you in the harness that cradles you safely and keeps you hooked up to the swing, or you'd have fallen off the toilet—and 'rung your bell' (i.e., hit your head), broken an arm, or worse, a hip.

Those with a prolapsed rectum (i.e., parts of their innards come out) enjoy the added discomfort of a nurse reinserting everything up your a-hole with their cold, gloved fingers.

After the paperwork, you're lifted back into your wheelchair. Now, the clock on three-day cycle starts all over again.

At least you didn't soil yourself, like two nights ago when you were incontinent of urine and woke up soaking wet. Who knows how long you'd been lying in bed like that?

Does soiling yourself because nobody can come fast enough feel right? Fair? Dignified?

But how can each person get the help they need to get to the toilet in time when there are thirty residents and four staff? Sounds like a complex, structural, procedural issue without a clear solution.

I'll take a medium coffee, hold the prunes, and make mine an extra-absorbent brief, please.

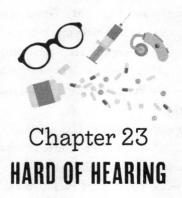

Chapter 23
HARD OF HEARING

It comes as no surprise that you can't fling a dead cat in a long-term care home without stumbling across a resident who is hard of hearing. Even with hearing aids in. Even with *their* hearing aids in. Without the batteries being dead, even.

Surprisingly, it isn't always the male residents who require hearing aids (from years of damaging their hearing on the job); you might otherwise have been forgiven for thinking it would have been skewed based on gender, but it's typically split quite evenly.

It goes without saying that communication can be, at times, rather... challenging, especially since roughly half of the staff are foreign-born with English as their second (or third ... or fourth) language. Imagine the resident's perspective: here you are, sitting in your wheelchair with the staff standing several feet above you, with (or without) *your* hearing aids in, trying to understand someone speaking with a thick accent, with a limited vocabulary, in a rush, likely wearing a mask ... while a lot of noise is blaring in the background.

Expecting clear, concise communication is like Hercules' brother: *Ridicules*. Didn't get that? Exactly the point.

Although it must be said that, understandably, some residents— very nearly all female—are too embarrassed (vain, perhaps?) to want to wear their hearing aids. The desire to look good in public doesn't fade (guessing that the beige tubes and bits are just too much and clash with the fifty-year-old earrings).

Doesn't mean to say that the clever ones can't still have some fun; playing with words and manipulating language can bring levity and comedic relief to almost any situation.

Take, for example, one resident who was fastidious about watching the news on CBC. Their TV was on nearly 24/7 with the volume set to 'rock concert' level (their door was schubsequently closed most of the time; at least the staff were always well informed of the latest events, as you could still hear live coverage from the other side of the unit). Their favourite news anchor was Ian Hanomansing—or, as they understood, Ian Handsomemanthing. We all knew when he was on because the TV's volume got turned up to *MAX*.

They are old, not dead. Their parts still work (well, except for their ears).

And speaking of parts still working, it is interesting to see how the hard of hearing are somewhat more disinhibited with respect to passing wind in public. Perhaps because they can't hear their own trumpeting misleads them into thinking nobody else can either. But we sure can. And we can all smell 'em.

You smelt it, you dealt it.

But don't for a moment write off all residents as senile; don't paint them all with the same brush. There are always silver linings, even to the crummiest of circumstances.

When asked how they're doing, some particularly challenged resi-dents (i.e., nearly deaf) offer a surprisingly positive outlook: *"I'm not*

hard of hearing. I'm just tired of listening to all the clap trap. Whenever I've
had enough of people, I just turn my hearing aids off."

Silence can be golden.

If only we could all unplug from the noise so easily.

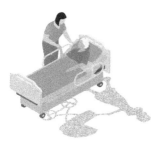

Chapter 24
TUBES

"Why does grandpa have so many tubes sticking out of him?"

This brings new meaning to being "well connected," although most in these circumstances would likely prefer not to be. There can be very little more humbling than getting to the point of requiring constant, visually-observable medical intervention to live normally – but that's the harsh reality of aging for many. It's funny how grounding it can be to have to re-examine our priorities in the face of illness; how nonsensical and trivial previous pre-occupations, vanities and concerns no longer are.

The reality is that many people in LTC have got themselves at least one tube. The "lucky" ones may have two . . . or three. As we age, stuff starts to function poorly, hence the need for a little help with either getting stuff out or putting stuff in—something for us all to look forward to.

And they all do something different.

Typically, the most frequent tube you'll see is a urinary catheter. So, gents, as I stated before, that means someone's got to insert a tube right up your old chap while you're awake and, usually, rather embarrassingly, all shrivelled up (*"I'm a grow-er, not a show-er, I swear!"*). Women, typically, don't have such a feeling of discomfort . . . once the tube goes into the right hole (new clinical staff often anticipate this potential error by having two catheters in tow – just in case their first attempt winds up in the vagina instead of urethra).

In one rather delicate example, a recently graduated nurse wasn't stopped by the resident from jabbing her clitoris repeatedly as she was attempting to insert the catheter. In fact, the resident let this go on for quite a while (much to the growing frustration and professional embarrassment of the nurse). At first, the nurse thought the resident was simply being patient but then realized *why* she was being so patient.

Oops! How vexatious.

Urinary catheters are a bit of a double-edged sword. On the one hand, they're required when people are retaining urine (i.e., can't pee on their own even though they feel they need to go); you don't want their bladder to rupture. Obviously. On the other hand, they're an opening (a "portal" in health-care parlance) that then makes acquiring a urinary tract infection (UTI)—among several possibilities—all the more likely. And you do see a lot of funky-looking pee: cloudy, with sediment, with puss, lumpy, milky, green, or bloody—you name it. It's like a handful of Skittles: all the colours of the rainbow.

On rounds one day, the RN was conferring with an RPN about a resident who was retaining urine. The PSWs overheard and remarked that nobody was retaining as much urine as them (they were so busy that they couldn't get themselves to the toilet).

One of those *funny-because-it's-true* moments.

Intravenous (IV) tubes are fairly well understood, having featured in every health-related comedy-drama since the dawn of TV. Usually hooked up in the front side of the bend in your arm (where it bends at the elbow) but also found at the top of the hand—basically, wherever there's a nice, big, juicy vein. These are used to administer anything from hydration (in people who haven't been consuming enough fluids, for whatever reason) or antibiotic therapy and other treatments.

Tubes coming out of someone's stomach or up their nose are used for feeding (high-protein and nutrient-rich feeding fluid). These are commonly referred to as G-tubes. Again, as with the hydration IV, these are found in residents (literally) who have problems eating (usually due to a difficulty with swallowing).

> **NOTE:** A G-tube is not to be confused with G-string. Also, where it is inserted into the abdomen is NOT the G-spot, as logical as that might seem. Be clear on these points; it'll save you considerable public embarrassment.

Some wounds produce lots of drainage. In these circumstances, you want to get the fluid out from the wound, so it can heal properly without any fluid getting trapped and forming an abscess (basically, a sac of pus or purulent fluid . . . which you don't want). Dressings on such wounds will be changed frequently, and this drainage can be encouraged either by a small tube or special gauze that helps to draw (or "wick") it out.

When it's wet and yellow, it's time to be changed. That's likely good life advice in a wider sense, applicable to most things.

Some people have what's called a colostomy. Put simply, this is a scenario where you don't poop out your butt any more. Instead, your poop comes out of a hole in your abdomen where the surgeon brought part of the intestine right out. So, over this hole, you essentially "glue" a bag to collect your farts and turds throughout the day. Naturally, you want to be proactive in emptying this bag; what you *don't want* is it "exploding."

Speaking of exploding. If you haven't pooped in days, you are likely lucky enough to be in line to receive a fleet enema: a nice (hopefully warm . . . if they're considerate) shot of fluid through a tube inserted up the bum to help get things moving along the "Hersey Highway."

At the end stage of life, when someone has been deemed to be receiving palliative care, they have a very small tube inserted just under the flesh, usually in their thigh, to receive pain medication. These tiny ports are called butterflies (just because of the shape of the wing-looking yellow bits sticking out each side that help keep them in position). They don't hurt at all, and it's the nicest way to provide someone with medication when they can't swallow (and likely don't want to be turned over to take something up the butt). Once inserted, a butterfly is a painless way to administer medication without sticking a needle into the resident every time (which can be as frequently as every hour). Someone may have a couple of butterflies; in this case, each ought to be labelled with what specific medication it is for.

If someone is prone to choking (again, likely due to difficulties swallowing) or is experiencing a bout where they are producing a lot of phlegm that they cannot clear independently, you may see a suction machine nearby. As the name suggests, this will be used by the RN if someone cannot breathe due to choking. What comes out can range from what they were last eating/drinking, to the thickest yellow-green snot you have ever seen . . . with the stringy consistency of a double-helping of mozzarella on your favourite slice, except with a very distinctive, nausea-inducing odour. Still, it's always a gratifying experience to clear someone's airway and see their anxiety evaporate the moment they can breathe again – even if only while they're wearing nasal prongs, getting oxygen at 2L/min.

Take a moment today to enjoy being able to breathe, swallow, pee, and poop independently. Being able to relieve yourself may be the closest thing to an orgasm once you're older.

Tubes may be a lifeline . . . but the most important connection old folks have is with people. Don't forget that. Call and visit them often. And try not to stare at the catheter bag hanging out the bottom of their pants.

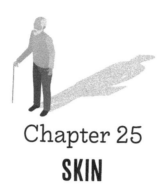

Chapter 25
SKIN

The integumentary system—our largest organ and the focus for a prolific beauty industry— continues to play an important part in long-term care, although not for the reasons you might suspect.

(Not that some of the older ladies don't still have a ritualistic routine of washing, removing makeup, and applying creams . . . old habits die hard. Besides, it's a good thing to take pride in your appearance. A ninety-year-old could easily be mistaken for looking at least ten years younger! And let's not discuss what those "cute" tattoos end up looking like fifty, sixty, seventy . . . years later.)

As we age, our skin and the supportive tissues directly beneath it, thin and lose their elasticity. Think of how thin the outer skin of an over-ripe tomato is. This is counter to what most people may assume—that wrinkly skin is somehow "tougher," and, well, it just isn't. That's a huge misnomer. As a result, considerable clinical attention is paid to monitoring the health and integrity of residents' skin.

Staff are always on the lookout for new (or seemingly enlarging) moles, skin tags, and dry or, more commonly, wet and cracking skin.

Skin breakdown from constant and unrelenting pressure (because people that can't move themselves any more can end up sitting in the same position for hours . . . think about that) or prolonged exposure to moisture (from being incontinent) are the most common culprits, causing skin breakdown and resulting ulcers (a wound where the skin opens up). Ulcers, if not treated, can be very serious with skin breaking down and dying off until bone is visible, at which point, regrowth will be almost impossible. Specialized, protective, barrier creams exist to prevent damage from moisture and to promote healing. Further, wound and skin dressings exist to wick moisture away and to provide additional padding and protective covering. Care staff will also be responsible for constant, regularly scheduled repositioning of residents who cannot move themselves—all in the name of keeping skin healthy. It's truly a multi-pronged approach, and prevention is the name of the game.

Not only are cuts, bruises, skin tears—all, unfortunately, common side effects from falls and slips—painful (and unsightly to look at), they open up a portal for infection. Even so little as sheering caused from clothing or blankets drawn on too tightly or quickly can become a pathway for infection.

Then you've got a whole additional layer of complications to treat. Bruises may look nasty and take ages to heal.

A lifetime of sun damage will be obvious . . . but good luck finding a resident who'd trade having "nicer" skin for all those memories. There's probably a wise life lesson in there somewhere.

Speaking of sunlight, why are so many residents provided with vitamin D instead of being assisted to spend time outside (in the protected courtyard area) on a deliberate and regular basis?!

Might improve their mood and boost their immune system too (so you could cut the antidepressant use down also; sounds like a win-win).

Naturally, healing of wounds or infection in any resident who has poor intake (i.e., isn't eating or drinking much, particularly nutrient- and protein-rich foods or supplements) or who suffers with advanced dementia (difficult to direct and unable to advocate for their care needs) is especially complicated and renders treatment all the more challenging.

> **FUN FACT:** One misconception that ought to be addressed is the origin of the "old-person smell." This is not due to a lack of hygiene; rather, it is a result, primarily, of the chemical breakdown of a by-product of the skin glands (the compound 2-nonenal tends to be found in higher concentrations in older adults' skin) and their interaction with the normal bacteria we all carry on our skin.

Imagine making "old- person smell" a thing of the past with a simple cream. What a great idea for a new, geriatric-focused, beauty skin care product. Just saying.

The other tangential—and thorny issue (literally)—are nails, particularly of the feet. It's easy to forget that talons are growing under those cute socks and slippers. Not only are nails sharp, (causing injury to others—including staff—and making shoes uncomfortable to wear) but residents often can't cut them themselves (or have other medical issues) and need professional help (which isn't always available frequently). Enter the podiatrist (aka chiropodist)—they are foot professionals.

So, next time you're in visiting your parent or grandparent, take a look at their finger and toe nails (are they cut or clean?), and check them for any new cuts or bruising. Never mind if they smell old—they can't help it. They are as you will be one day. Ask if they'd like a little shuffle or help with a slight repositioning.

They'll appreciate feeling more comfortable in their own skin.

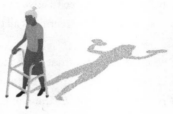

Chapter 26
STAFFING

"It's never a good sign when you pull into work at 5:40AM and the parking lot is suspiciously empty. Looks like I'll be working short again today. Fuck."

Okay. Please sit down, take a deep breath, and bear with me on this one. I'm trying to advance an argument here.

Skilled staffing sounds easy, but in practice, it rarely comes off without several hitches. The need to staff the organization adequately and appropriately is a full-time job in and of itself. With fifty or more staff on at any moment, making sure every position is filled given the constant flux of sick calls, vacation days, orientation of new staff and modified duties of those requiring accommodation is a daunting logistical challenge.

Soft skills are essential to succeed. Honestly, you need a PhD in common sense, human and organizational psychology, modern languages, strategic planning, economics, cost containment, patience, social work, multitasking, and negotiation (i.e., combination of manipulative techniques and grovelling) to make sense of it all, let alone to make any progress. Add in the fact that you're working with people (and not machines), so layers of misunderstandings, office politics, and feelings only complicate matters further; indeed, tell me what your problem is and I'll make it more difficult.

To be clear (and fair), we need to distinguish between culpable and non-culpable absenteeism. The latter are appropriate (i.e. when people are genuinely ill, the last place they should be is work); it's all the inappropriate examples of the former that we need to tackle.

A simple sick call can take hours to fill—if that is even possible to do so within the constraints of time, union-imposed, seniority-based calling order, and inconsistent support by management to offer to pay overtime (OT; usually paid at one and a half times the normal rate of pay). This inconsistency can backfire because staff might decline to work at regular pay, instead electing to take an educated gamble that OT will then be offered. It usually is. Often, someone will pick up (only at OT rate, obviously) and then stipulate the condition that they will do the OT only if they are afforded a day off later. So, you're no further ahead (when do you want to be short: now or later?) but are so indebted to them and desperate in the moment that you have no option but to accept (it's the marginal utility of the offer that matters; i.e., how badly do you need *this* RPN on *this* day on *this* unit on *this* shift?!). Indeed, staffers have to keep an accurate mental ledger to balance the needs of today with those down the road. Understand the basic truth that availability (and willingness) to work is the coin of the realm. Being beholden to and bedevilled by the few who step up is a currency they can trade in. And they know it.

The price of an unfilled shift does not fully capture the true cost of the vacancy (the detriment to others can be profound). Such is the externality. The proclivity of people to stick it to their peers by being chronically absent never fails to dumbfound me; it's as if they're ensconced in a broader moral framework that simply accepts culpable absenteeism as normal (encouraged, even).

How OT is approved or distributed may depend also on who the leader on call is on the day. . . and how badly they don't want to come in to cover the staff vacancy themselves (the more they want to avoid doing so, the higher the chance they'll approve OT). It's all a game, and to "win," you have to know the players. After hours, the responsibility of staffing often falls to the RN on duty because . . . *why not?!*

Casual observations: Often, OT will not be approved unless a manager has to come in to cover the shift (or unless there's other "special" grant funding available—then spend as much as you want! They'll offer OT like a PEZ dispenser). Having to cover a night shift is the most common example where inconsistencies (i.e., staffing policy based on convenience) are rife. For example, the on-call manager might not grant OT to cover an RPN's evening shift (thereby reducing the chances of anyone accepting the shift from nearly zero to absolutely zero). As a consequence, the RN will have to work short and cover a unit in addition to their other responsibilities. Then, when the night RN calls in sick, the same on-call manager will beg the evening RN to extend (i.e., to work sixteen hours) to cover the night shift, so the manager doesn't have to come in. Now, that same manager is asking a favour from the very person they just screwed over. This isn't uncommon.

In unionized environments, the collective agreements dictate that staff must be called in a particular order (typically by seniority within full-time, part-time or casual status); otherwise, members can submit a grievance. (If they win, they are paid for the shift they didn't work; ensuring that the order of seniority is observed perfectly adds another dimension and slows the entire call-out process). Never mind the fact that those who grieve are typically the ones who decline to come in any time they're asked but still make damn sure they are called every time. Interestingly, it's always curious to observe how many people can't receive a new voicemail when called to come in because their *"inbox is full."* How many calls result in a full voicemail inbox?! Consistently?!

Makes you shake your head.

It's not uncommon for units to run short of staff for consecutive shifts—simultaneously. Multiple sick calls (i.e., well into the double-digits) per day are not unusual (well, except on stat holidays, of course, where everyone is paid at the OT rate, so they all come in). On beautiful summer evenings, it's as if "Dr. Summeroff" has been busy writing notes to excuse a suspiciously high number of people from work. Ensuring the building is adequately staffed can feel like trying to solve a Rubik's Cube that's fighting back: nothing is more frustrating than *finally* patching together coverage for a gap only to have another call come in. And then another. Moreover, people who simply don't show up for their scheduled shift without even notifying anyone beforehand (and who schubsequently don't return calls to ask if they're coming in) are not uncommon.

Management take heed: *What you permit, you promote.* Do not tolerate no-shows. Crack down stridently and quickly on such irresponsible and selfish behaviours. I'm emphatic about this because I've seen the damage it does to staff morale and how it contributes to the poorer care outcomes that are suffered when working short—especially when it becomes predictable, and there seems to be no consequences for irresponsible absenteeism (and therefore, no discernable rationale for being responsible and coming in). Absenteeism is infectious. It's a negative spiral brought on by the following positive feedback loop: the more people work short, the more they call in sick, and the more people who call in sick, the more others work short, and so on and so forth.

If not addressed, this can become a self-fulfilling prophecy and an entrenched mentality (that it's simply okay and accepted practice to call in simply because you don't want to work). In the end, when their truant counterparts' behaviours aren't managed appropriately, the good staff are those who are punished (not only by working short but also by having their vacation or mutually-agreed shift-trade requests denied—perhaps due to a lack of necessary coverage to backfill their leave). So, now, you have a scenario where a loyal and conscientious staff member becomes conflicted; they need time off, but if they apply for it appropriately, they know the request will be denied . . . so they're left with no alternative but to call in sick.

And downward goes the spiral. All to the detriment of the entire organization's culture.

Yet, there are a few examples that are clearly 'wrong' but to which you are sympathetic... which leave you frustrated and torn. For instance, can you blame a young employee, in their early 20s, who are late to work (scheduled 7:00 AM start) because they were up until 3:00 AM at their other job? But what if they *need* that other job to log the requisite hours for their Canadian citizenship application? Can you really get mad at them when they sleep in? Repeatedly? No easy answer.

Perhaps leadership ought to consider the strategic value of offering a bonus to any employee who wants to quit; let them self-select out of the organization—passive pruning. Good riddance.

. . . or maybe not. Might be too much to stomach. Best to apply a monthly cap to slow the exodus until you've got the new hires fully trained.

As progressive as it might sound to offer a bonus to any employee who refers someone who then applies and is hired, there ought to be investigative questions posed when nobody follows through on the incentive. It's likely a highly correlative proxy for low organizational morale. Might be worth looking into and addressing the root causes.

It's fascinating to observe that the Pareto principle never fails: it seems that it's always the same 20 percent of staff who call in "sick" 80 percent of the time; moreover, it's a different 20 percent of staff who will work extra 80 percent of the time to pick up their slack (*Must be tough being young and "sick" all the time, eh?*). Further, why there remains any local unemployment whatsoever boggles the mind; anyone willing to work (maybe *that's* the issue) could easily find an opportunity at their local LTC home, I'd venture. Perhaps the city should erect signs at the closest main intersection to each home or pay someone to wear one of those crazy fuzzy suits and dance with a sign to point them in the right direction for employment opportunities.

At this moment, I'd like to point out that the same OT rate of pay can be earned almost every day (given the volume and consistency of sick calls)—not just on stat holidays—if people just wanted to work.

As a litmus test for the organization's internal political health, it's remarkable to watch which units are unsettled, when, and why. The intuitive predictive value of a veteran staff member's foresight of who might call in and when is eerily accurate. Often, a unit will place its own interests over their neighbouring unit (because each unit believes *it's busier than everyone else, don't you know*) and not be forthcoming about if they are fully staffed or, by some miracle, have an extra staff member. Games are rife. Units with the most staff will complain that they need more. A unit that is short will complain incessantly (ironically, the person doing the complaining is often the one who calls in "sick" the most often; see the Pareto principle above), even after it has been explained that every avenue has been taken to support them. A personal favourite of mine is when a unit that is running short (and made it known in no uncertain terms) *declines* help.

You can't suck and blow. Give your head a shake. Seriously. Are you really *that* obtuse? Is it deliberate?!

As brevity is the soul of wit, here are some head-scratching examples of the types of scenarios beset by those charged with solving staffing problems (problems that often shouldn't exist):

Six female staff call in (strangely, within minutes of each other) citing painful menstrual cramps for the same shift (talk about synchronizing their cycles). One put it particularly vividly: *"My vagina won't stop bleeding!"*

Guess it must have been shark week. And not just on the Discovery Channel.

A support worker presents themself for work with self-described respiratory symptoms during an outbreak and is "surprised" they are turned away. When asked why they didn't call in sick, they respond, *"They love the residents."*

Dipshit.

From a staffing perspective, there are three interesting coincidences with this example: it's the nicest day of the year; the worker is retiring at the end of the month and had had vacation booked for this day that had schubsequently been rescinded on account of the outbreak and enhanced staffing requirements. As stated already, a staff member who is denied a vacation request (because there isn't anyone available to cover while they are off) may resort to calling in "sick" for that same shift.

Or how about when a staff member calls in, and it's a beautiful summer's day, or it's their birthday (as due to Facebook, everyone happens to know), and they provide only one symptom that just happens to be not outbreak-related (i.e., *"I have a sore back"*) and is impossible to dispute? I'm sure they hope we're to believe this is all mere coincidence.

For kicks, here are some other examples of juicy excuses:

"I've got the worst UTI! It's like I'm pissing needles."

"I can't come into work. I've got an ingrown toenail."

"My cat's sick. I couldn't possibly make it in."

"I've got a flat tire. I just can't take a cab, bus, or Uber to get there at any point in the next twelve hours."

"I know I picked up the overtime shift, but I'm tired and don't want to do it anymore." This passive-aggressive behaviour results in hogging the OT and thereby preventing someone else from accepting (and from working) the shift. Naturally, it's then next to impossible to find a replacement with no notice.

"Do you have a line now?" (i.e., Do you have a regular, bi-weekly schedule?) *"Yes, on Hibiscus unit; that's why I'm scheduled for Tulip and working on Dandelion."* Confused? This provides a glimpse to the

chaotic nature of staffing—not knowing necessarily where you're going to be working despite supposedly having a set schedule, as it all depends on the particular demands of the day (and who's shown up).

But hey, if you do pick up an extra shift, make sure to wear your cape when you come in because you're a superhero saving the day.

Another interesting observation is that floors have become conditioned to keeping their mouths shut in the event they are fully staffed; when you're fully staffed, you "can't expect it to last long" before someone is pulled to help cover another unit. Staffing woes (too common and never addressed) include no show, no call, no callback, no consequences, and no improvement. An enlightened management team might do well to consider staffing to be *the* one target problem where upstream investment would pay the most profound dividends (i.e., would lower financial costs to the organization and generate higher staff morale and better care of residents). Yet, this is the one facet where the downstream epitome of fly-by-the-seat-of-your-pants approach (i.e., lean on your most dedicated/burned-out employees to save the day—again) is taken perennially.

Leaders, by addressing chronic staffing vacancies quickly, proactively, and visibly (i.e. communicating that you are doing so), you're essentially saying: "I hear you," and you're acknowledging the plight of those who demonstrate the integrity of being present regularly in spite of working short. Besides, advocating for employees who are poorly positioned to influence the system that results in them being short-handed will address the pejorative feelings of hopelessness and loss-of-control that erode their organizational commitment and morale.

In my opinion, the principle of Occam's razor is sound and relevant, as usual. Recognize that common things are common. Reduce the argument to its core while excising all unnecessary distractions, excuses, and red herrings. The simplest explanation and underlying reason to most problems is attributable to a lack of adequate staffing.

Know anyone looking for a job?

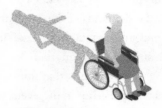

Chapter 27
LET'S SQUARE THE CIRCLE

After the previous chapter on staffing, I didn't want you to think I was on my soapbox having a good moan. . . . At least, I didn't want you to think that was *all* that I was doing. So, best to bring some (*very* basic) statistical methodology to the party. Let's shoot for the moon and attempt to square the circle. After all, if you're not part of the solution, you're part of the problem.

And I've been at the receiving end of this problem for too long not to venture a solution or two. (These are among the things I'm trying to solve mentally with thought experiments when I'm a 17.62/10 grump-asaurus from working short.)

We need to establish and agree that, in large part, staffing and hiring are, in essence, a judgment call. That's the premise here. Therefore, it stands to reason that as with any human-based decision, it's subject to biases, errors, and inconsistencies. Not to mention pesky scheduling conflicts and delays. It's a messy process rife with irregularities and waste. So, how can we work around these shortfalls?

Enter the staffing/hiring algorithm.

Sacrilege?! Isn't human involvement and engagement in hiring sacrosanct?!

Bull crackers.

Humans are, in fact, the weak link in the chain. Besides, using even a simple algorithm during the hiring process should return better results more quickly and cheaply—not to mention that algorithms are blind to race, religion, gender, etc. The results are objectively based on the merit of the inputs. To understand more accurately how much can be saved, hiring managers (as well as anyone else involved in interviews) need to account for the value of the time they spend on the hiring process as a cost—in addition to the advertising budget spent. The amount of wasted time (i.e., money) and lost productivity are not always apparent when you're on salary . . . but we'll gloss over that inconvenient truth for the time being.

"But what if I'm 'uncomfortable' adopting a computer or an algorithm?" Would it help if we called it a supportive "hiring tool questionnaire" instead? Maybe even give it a name? Let's call it Joel; he sounds clever. Would that make it . . .errr, "him" more trustworthy?

If that's what you need to tell yourself to take a leap of faith—then yes, yes it does. (Sometimes you gotta say: *"What the fuck"* and make your move.)

Even the most ponderous, bureaucratic, and intransigent organizations can implement something so simple reasonably quickly (i.e., after fewer than half-a-dozen committee meetings).

So, to be clear, the goal here is to create a simple questionnaire that candidates can complete themselves and submit (it's not like mild fibbery and embellishments don't happen in traditional interviews already). The hiring team can then score each application (the final tally simply being the total sum of the questions' responses; say, each question is scored on a one to five Likert scale) and simply rank them from lowest to highest (the higher number, the better)—all without clapping eyes on the applicants.

First, anyone looking to hire needs to spend deliberate time and focus wording the job description for the vacant position as clearly, thoroughly, and honestly as possible. How well this is completed reflects on the hiring organization. Moreover, don't post anything generic; if you're looking for night-shift coverage, say so accurately. Let people self-regulate and not bother applying if they aren't interested (and don't be surprised when people who wanted days or evenings leave when all they're offered are nights). Being both honest and trust-worthy is two-way street; be upfront with what you want and what you don't. Another classic example is when people want a full-time posi-tion but are only offered part-time (or casual) and then, once hired, are called for additional shifts totalling at least full-time hours. Again, like trust, if you won't commit to an employee, they won't commit to you; hire as many full-time people as you can so that you do not lose them to other employers (i.e., do not waste all the invested time and money spent in their orientation). The additional investments associated with this approach will pay dividends.

Let's take the example of hiring PSWs (but this could be applied to almost any position in LTC). The primary goal is to find candidates who will demonstrate consistently higher rates of attendance (never mind that attendance is also a welcome proxy of conscientiousness—another key trait of successful hires, as it speaks to discretionary effort and level of skill). The second goal, as is current practice, is to set the minimum standards for someone to be considered a candidate. The best example is education; they need to have completed the necessary training successfully to apply for the job. Other criteria may be to dem-onstrate a clean criminal record, up-to-date vaccination status (as well as absence of reportable communicable diseases; i.e., active pulmonary TB), or perhaps you may require that they possess a current driver's license. These are all binary, simple, yes–no questions; a single "no" would exclude them from further consideration. Add to this list as you see fit.

These "mechanical" requirements make intuitive sense and can be confirmed before the next step in the interview process. They are reasonable and part of current hiring practice. Nothing new thus far.

Third, you should decide what the qualities of a successful hire and long-term employee are. To not have a good sense of this from the outset is nothing short of risky business: like pissing into the wind, it'll come back to get you.

In the land of statistics, it is said that you "do not need models more precise than your measurements." So, don't expect your first kick at the algorithm to be perfect. You can refine it over time until you come across a set of questions that fits your organization's goals and culture.

Remember, all you need is a set of predictors that correlate with the desired outcome; the score of each question posed manages an important quality(ies) required for success. You need to determine the questions to ask in order to set the bar high enough; all you need are people who are good *enough,* not outliers (by definition, they're rare). Be comfortable not knowing if someone will work out or not once hired—that's what the probationary period is for. Extend it if necessary.

Fourth is to adopt a simple, equal weight model where each question is equivalently influential to the overall candidate's summed score (also implied is that the difference between each question's rating is the same; i.e., the difference between one and two is as great as between four and five). This is important because it means that shortcomings in one area will average out with strengths in another (rather than the subjective preponderance of human adjudicators to overaccentuate or de-emphasize aspects in order to fit their personal, inconsistent biases). This way, as the popular saying goes, the whole trick is to "know which variables to look at . . . and to know how to add." Let the invisible hand of the algorithm take it from there.

Such a simple model will, in the long run, do nearly as well as a more complex statistical model (i.e., weighted average least squares), will outperform case-by-case human judgment almost certainly, and is faster, cheaper, and reproducible (regardless of the people involved on either side). If you assume the realistic perspective that your organization will incur 10 to 20 percent (conservative estimate) staff turnover per annum, you're looking to hire at least twenty people every year. Can you start to see how much time you'll save and how many candidates you can sort through quickly? Think of the number of days a vacant position goes unfilled currently; I'd wager there's much room for improvement. Besides, hiring qualified people faster benefits everyone and will result in higher employee satisfaction scores . . . and better care outcomes . . . and less overtime . . . and less "sick" time.

I'm not advocating abandoning traditional interviews . . . entirely (managers still need to spend time getting to know their staff, to offer considered praise and specific feedback, and to set expectations, etc.). Rather, I'm highlighting that there's an "industrial" approach that could achieve results at least as good as current processes more efficiently. Define what success looks like and select questions accordingly. Then, shift the emphasis and burden of responsibility from (delaying) hiring to focus on candidate performance management during the probationary period. Fail forward instead of paralysis by analysis.

Important disclaimer: do not misinterpret that I'm commoditizing people. I do *not* believe people are a dime-a-dozen; I know better than most how important devoted and honest employees are. All we're trying to do is to find these great staff members in a fresh and improved way.

Ultimately, to accept this new approach, you must be comfortable with:

- not meeting people first (i.e., selecting candidates to hire literally blindly); and
- trusting that data are often more trustworthy than personal judgement calls.

Algorithms make mistakes but fewer in the long run than humans; trust the data more than the preferences and beliefs of those tasked with hiring.

Indeed, time to start the interview process (perhaps it ought to be called "application process" instead) with a blank set of objective questions instead of the traditional subjective (and supremely unhelpful) ones, such as *"Describe your ideal day on the job"* *"What's your best quality?"* *"What's your worst quality (i.e., stop telling me that you're a perfectionist)?"* etc.

Some examples, for illustrative purposes only, of the types of objective questions that might be included on a questionnaire are:

- How many days did you miss class/work per month on average last year?
- How far away do you live from work?
- How many jobs have you had in last ten years? Since you graduated?
- How many times have you moved in the last ten years?
- How many times have you been promoted?
- How many years ago did you graduate? (Or, in what year did you graduate?)[4]

Most predictors are themselves related, so you can be more frugal than you first expected. Lean into the discomfort—it's all part of the process. Remember, a candidate's past behaviour is the strongest indicator of their future performance. Therefore, if they demonstrated a high absenteeism rate with respect to prior life commitments, they

---

4   Consider that the number of years since you graduated is a reasonable proxy for age (which you're *not* allowed to ask) and also how "hungry" the person will likely be to be present and pick up overtime.

will tend to recidivate. And yes, I'm suggesting that a simple calculation of two or three questions will likely paint a reasonably accurate picture of their risk to commit certain behaviours in the future (like frequent absenteeism).

Now, all you need to do is accept the number of candidates required to fill current vacancies who meet your mechanical questions and threshold score. Easy. As previously mentioned, don't worry about "soft" or "people" skills or the ever subjective "organizational fit" at this point; let people go who show insufficiency in these areas (and a lack of potential to improve) throughout the probationary period. BUT be fair and transparent; give advanced warnings and sufficient critical feedback, so candidates know what (and how) to develop while they still have chance to do so. Again, this approach will provide an opportunity for them to reveal how agreeable, amenable to feedback, and motivated they really are—thereby providing tremendous insight into the amount of discretionary effort and global conscientiousness they'll likely continue to demonstrate throughout their tenure.

Take it a step further, and you could create "equal" teams based on individual employee scores and balance out each unit on each shift. In the end, it's all about first getting the right people on the proverbial bus, then sitting them in the right seats.

Once you've finally got all your vacancies filled, there could be a place (although far less "needed") to adopt a tech-based solution for filling daily vacancies. For example, why isn't there readily (i.e., cheap) available software wherein you plug in all the algorithmic type of staff required, union-based calling order, overtime, vacation, leave parameters, etc., and then have it auto-dial voicemails, text message blast-out, and/or social media posts/direct messages? Why is it still up to a person to make one call after another (and to sit there listening to one person's voicemail message after another because nobody actually picks up when they see that it's work calling)?

To me, this description congers up an image of a 1960s-era lifelong secretary, Mrs. Blankenslop, dialling away on her rotary phone from a list written in fountain pen. . . as she's got a cigarette dangling from her lips, her cat eye glasses on point. Does this picture help describe how archaic our typical procedure remains?!

And if you *really* can't go with such a tool (*still too uncomfortable?*), the next best option would be to conduct all interviews over the phone. Avoid face-to-face interviews to the greatest degree possible; they are too distracting and don't actually provide any objective information that can't be obtained in 'blind' conversation (if anything, this approach may mitigate any confirmation biases that exist among the interviewer(s) and force deliberate attention be paid to perfect the interview questionnaire). Learn by listening to your candidates; it will be apparent how intelligent, conscientious, honest, kind, agreeable, selfless, and motivated they are.

That's all you need.

As a replacement for traditional interviews, an infallible tech-based solution would be cheaper, faster, non-judgmental, incontestable, and error-free—what a great idea for a business, product, or patient. Just saying. *Deus ex machina.*

I'm no quant or polymath (despite a rather "diverse" educational background and rich, assorted set of work experiences), but I can see the clear value-add of such a paradigm shift. Embrace the rise of the machines.

It's a good thing to be open-minded; questions challenge mindsets and can clear the way to find new solutions to old problems.

Never mind the fact that it would free up a registered nurse to be . . . a nurse, not a staffing clerk. I'm sure the residents would appreciate a clinician spending more time with them instead of on a rotary phone. And for that, there is no substitute.[5]

---

5   Those most fond of the old school *luftgekühlt* or Gmunds will get the reference.

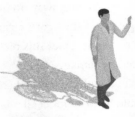

Chapter 28
OUTBREAKS

In coordination with the local Public Health authorities, LTC homes (as would any hospital unit, jail, retirement, or group homes, etc.) monitor their resident population at the group level. This is to say, are there any emerging trends where multiple people are coming down with the same constellation of symptoms simultaneously? If so, the sooner action can be taken to stop the spread and/or identify a causative agent, the less severe the outcomes and the shorter the duration of the outbreak itself. The precautionary principle demands quick, decisive action to decrease the risk of spread of an infectious agent (in a vulnerable population) in order to prevent an outbreak – prudence with purpose; however, if ever measures seem like an over-reaction, they are not meant to be punitive. Remember, outcomes are rarely in anyone's control; processes are.

Public Health authorities act as a resource for best practices with respect to surveillance requirements, pathogen identification, outbreak declaration, and consult on schubsequent interventions intended to curtail spread and identify the fastest possible path to outbreak resolution. All best practices are science-based; however, the implementation of measures highlight the fact that outbreak management is both a science and an art. In LTC homes, you are working with multiple people, twenty-four hours a day, some of whom are confused and wander when they ought to remain isolated, and most rooms share a common bathroom. See the inherent problems?

Indeed, there are both positive and negative externalities that must be balanced throughout outbreak management as a result of the significant control measures which must be implemented.

For example, it is completely understandable that loving family members become distraught at the prospect of having their visiting privileges curtailed or suspended temporarily during an outbreak, but the intentions here are both to protect the residents from outside exposures and those coming in from taking home what's known to be circulating. It can feel punitive, but it isn't meant to be. For families anxious to keep in touch with their older parents during these times, one strategy might be to work with the care team to arrange phone calls or virtual meetings. This will ensure phone calls aren't missed and residents are ready on time.

It must be said that infection control is truly a shared responsibility; it only takes one slip (by anyone) to transmit an infectious agent (i.e., the visitor who fails to wash their hands . . . after using the bathroom; this happens, so don't be offended if you're reminded to wash your hands frequently when visiting). But if staff and visitors do their part correctly, benefits spill out and protect everyone.

NOTE: When "shopping around" for an LTC home, an interesting question to pose to the staff is the frequency/number of outbreaks that occur in a typical year. This will provide keen insight into how effective the global functioning of the home may be. For example, how well do management collaborate with Public Health? How well engineered is the building itself? How well trained are the staff? How available is the necessary PPE? How few (or many) people may be isolated at any given time? Etc.

Staff don't need to be reminded of the importance of wearing proper personal protective equipment (PPE) and frequent and deliberate handwashing (nobody enjoys the "salmonella weight loss diet" however effective it may be). But the continuous donning and doffing of gloves, gowns, masks, goggles, and booties, the endless application of hand sanitizer, and so on does become labourious and slows down the ability to jump from one resident to the next. Patience is indeed a virtue, and so is the ability to tolerate getting all dolled up and working in the oppressive heat and humidity of the summer. It's draining and unpleasant. But it's the sacrifice made for the utilitarian greater good (with positive externalities to an incalculable multiple of people).

Interestingly, those of the eco-friendly mindset would be best to turn a blind eye at the amount of waste created by single-use PPE disposed of in health-care facilities, particularly during outbreaks, not to mention the cleaning chemicals. Just saying.

The downsides to being in outbreak are difficult to qualify as the major unintended consequence to anyone placed in isolation (twenty-four hours, forty-eight hours, ten days, two weeks—totally depends on the underlying bug) is the understandable boredom, loneliness, and perceived lack of attention/care (how would you feel if you weren't "allowed" to come out of your room for days on end?!). The staff are acutely aware of how unpleasant it must feel and how challenging it is to maintain. Good-natured remarks by clinical staff to asymptomatic residents still in isolation add much-needed comedic relief, *"I see you're still in the slammer, eh, Marlene? Have you run out of toilet paper yet?"* Always worth a laugh.

The tricky part comes in being as fair and balanced as possible with respect to who must go into isolation in the first place. You want to place the right people in isolation for the right reason and for the right duration of time—and nobody else. There are subtle nuances to being in isolation and of outbreak management—this is why outbreak management is both a science and an art.

So, for example, let's say there has been an enteric (stomach bug) outbreak declared (think how much fun it will be to collect the poop samples and then "place" them into containers . . . and then label them . . . and then drive them to the lab yourself—screw the lid on *tight!*) and friendly Helen has only just had a large, loose BM after not having gone for three days (which is actually pretty normal for her).

Because she hadn't been going, she'd been receiving ever more frequent (and potent) motility agents and stool softeners, so she had become akin to a powder keg that was bound to explode at some point. No other symptoms. Yet, by the outbreak definitions, she ought to be isolated as a precautionary measure—is that right? Fair? Not to mention the fact that her roommate (also completely asymptomatic), by definition (because they share a room and a bathroom, thus considered co-infected), must now be isolated, too.

Double whammy (and hence the "value" of obtaining a private room, if at all possible).

> **LESSON:** If you can afford it, it's worth paying the extra for a private room.

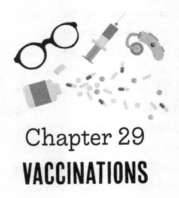

Chapter 29
VACCINATIONS

Always best to keep the communicable diseases at bay, especially in vulnerable (and captive— literally) populations. Prevention is key.

Upon admission, a full medical history will be taken (hopefully with background documents forwarded on from the most recent family physician). Vaccination history and status will be a focus; the more accurate and complete a resident's records, the better. Have them handy. Most residents are due for booster shots at some point (e.g., Adacel for tetanus-diphtheria-pertussis). You might be interested to learn that the local Public Health authority monitors the temperatures of any fridge in LTC that contains vaccines to ensure that everything is maintained within safe limits. A vaccine is as likely to spoil (and, thus, needs to be discarded) if it is stored at too cold a temperature as it is if not kept cold enough. Generally speaking, freezing vaccines guarantees they're going straight in the trash instead of into someone's arm; what you want to avoid is administering inoculations that have been rendered inert—they will not offer any protection.

Residents will be required to prove they do not have active tuberculosis (TB) in a part(s) of the body that would render them contagious before they can be admitted—for obvious reasons. This will result in everyone being required to have a chest X-ray or a sputum sample (spit/hork sample) come back clear (negative) before admission to LTC can proceed. TB skin tests are generally less reliable as we age, so while a negative TB test may be a criterion for employees and volunteers, it likely won't be for residents.

Families, or anyone responsible for giving consent for medical treatment, will be asked by the care team for consent on a yearly basis before administering seasonal influenza (or COVID-19) shots or preventive treatments like antivirals (e.g., Tamiflu) in the event an outbreak is declared in collaboration with the local Public Health authority. At the same time, any boosters that may be due will be confirmed and consent obtained. Discussions regarding vaccination status against pneumococcal, shingles, and tetanus-diphtheria-pertussis are especially pertinent in older adults.

Traditionally, from the staff perspective, there has always been a decision to be made about getting the yearly flu shot (i.e., get the shot or be required to wear a mask). Even then, the non-vaccinated staff may not be permitted to work should there be an outbreak declared—and in seasons where there's a mismatch between circulating strains and those in the shot, everyone will be obligated to wear a mask anyway. Naturally, since the pandemic, anyone in a health-care facility will have had to submit for testing on a regular and frequent basis (so don't complain about having a swab shoved up your nose once—we've had to do it repeatedly for months).

After a particularly deeply irritating and uncomfortably ticklish nasopharyngeal swab (i.e., the type that make your eyes water and induce a cough-sneeze reaction), the receiving RN joked that it was reassuring to learn that they managed to survive the '80s with their nasal septum intact.

Nobody in the room got the joke. Never mind. They were all too young.

Let's not forget Rufus either. If you are planning to have your (approved) pet come in, make sure they're all up to date too. Don't need ticks or fleas about the place. People are itchy enough as it is.

And for the elephant in the quagmire of the perennial debate: Being a "conscientious objector" to being vaccinated will cause friction and additional challenges, particularly during outbreaks. While everyone may be required to wear PPE (gloves, gown, and mask) when in the building regardless, please consider that you are putting yourself and others at (avoidable) risk. That's why they are called "vaccine preventable" diseases—VPDs.

No judgement or shame. Just a fact.

Please remember to follow these basic *Rules of Infection Control for All Time:*

- Wash your hands thoroughly and frequently, especially after using the bathroom, changing a baby, touching an animal, and before preparing and eating food. Use soap and water and rub vigorously for as long as it takes to sing *Happy Birthday*.
- Observe proper coughing and sneezing etiquette (i.e., into the elbow of your sleeve).
- If you're sick, stay home.
- Wash and cook your food thoroughly.
- Get vaccinated.

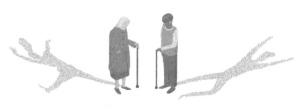

Chapter 30
THE FOOD

Mmmm. Nomm nomm nomm nomm nomm.

It's quite the logistical feat to feed over 150 residents three meals and multiple snacks each day across one main kitchen and multiple serveries (usually one per unit or floor). And that's assuming "the kitchen" is fully staffed—which it often isn't. Not to mention the precautions that must be made to accommodate for individual requirements (e.g., allergies, specific textures, etc.). Public Health has their say also, and each home's kitchen is subject to routine inspection for cleanliness, food-handling practices, correct storage, proper temperature control, and appropriate washing techniques.

Mealtimes tend to become the "next event" in the otherwise monotonous day, often with residents lining up to get into the communal dining room (sometimes up to an hour before mealtime) because there's nothing else to do. It is a social event, well, for some, anyway (e.g., two residents would refuse anyone who dared to sit at their table, believing they were cognitively superior, yet they would repeat the identical conversation every time they ate together—intellect and memory are two different things).

Interestingly, some residents couldn't be more disinterested in the food or the social atmosphere (like Marjorie, who always got her best sleep in the dining room at breakfast time until she woke herself up after a particularly shrill, nasal snore). It's not uncommon for residents to give their food away to others sitting around them. While *sharing is caring*, the dangers of being given food not otherwise intended can bring with it complications relating to allergies and unsafe consistencies to those at risk for choking.

Credit where credit is due: the PSW staff develop incredible memories for residents' food preferences (much like taxi drivers in London, England, develop enlarged hippocampi as they train for "The Knowledge"). Without blinking an eye, most are able to recall the individual drink preference and preparation, food consistency, room number and location, and any special utensils for twenty or more residents. Perfectly. Every time.

It's uncanny.

And this is important. In an environment where most residents have some degree of difficulty swallowing, serving food at the wrong consistency could result in undue risk for choking. It may seem trivial, but knowing the difference between minced or pureed foods or how thick to serve fluids is *really* critical (there's usually a suction machine in each dining room in the event someone's airway gets blocked—and there needs to be).

Not that you can necessarily tell what the food was before it was mushed up.

NOTE: Metaphorically speaking, we tend cut up people's 'food' for them so much, they've stopped being able to think and reason for themselves whereas the onus remains on all families and/or substitute decision-makers to be informed, responsible and available.

During outbreaks, when residents are separated and eat alone—making it more difficult to supervise adequately—the risk for people choking becomes even greater. While safety is considered of utmost importance, it must be said, it often comes at the expense of gastronomic pleasure. Does the thought of "drinking" thickened, room-temperature water or not being able to recognize what you're about to eat among three heaps of pureed food (every meal, everyday) sound appetizing?! No wonder mealtimes can take over an hour. Blagh!

Interestingly, a resident who complains about the food (*"What's this? A bologna sandwich on white bread on Christmas Day?!"*) is just as likely to then ask for more. And promptly forget they've eaten as soon as they leave the dining room, only to complain that nobody is feeding them. Funny in a sad-bad sort of way.

There are a variety of modified eating utensils to facilitate independence at mealtimes. For example, plates with higher lips or cups with two handles enable residents greater leverage. Foam handles to facilitate grip (for arthritic hands that can't clasp tightly) or bent cutlery (like what you might find in a Salvador Dali painting) facilitate the process of moving food from plate to mouth. Often, there will be a handful of residents who cannot feed themselves and must therefore wait their turn (a PSW will sit in between two residents and feed them at once while in the dining room). Hopefully, their pureed food is at least still warm. Hopefully.

Once, one resident, while being fed in the dining room, suffered a fatal stroke, convulsed, and slumped over—all in less than five seconds. Out. Gone. Dead. We didn't tell the chef.

Unfortunately, there seem to be few dietary choices for vegetarians or vegans (as often pointed out by staff who follow such diets). Overall, residents are usually fed lower-quality, high-carb food, and sugary snacks (and we wonder why people's teeth rot, particularly given poor oral care) and, over time, gain unhealthy weight (fat) as a consequence.

Families who request that their parent be given "ginger ale" because their stomach is upset should realize that it doesn't actually contain any ginger (it's just the cheapest stuff you can buy . . . obviously). Sadly, the per resident, per diem budget can be roughly on par with that for those in some correctional facilities (the irony that both populations could be considered incarcerated isn't lost). That's what can happen when homes are privately owned; not every aspect of our publicly funded health-care system is . . . publicly funded. Most are surprised to learn this. (In fact, most long-term care homes are privately owned.)

Of course, a few families do their best to bring in food (or coffee!) from home for their parent or friend. This is a treat—it's really the simple things in life that make the difference. The supply line is often rendered more challenging during outbreaks. Famously, one family placed meatballs in an envelope and same-day couriered them in—as is often the case, where there is a will, there is a way.

Snoring folk, a choke, a stroke, and mailed in meatballs . . . it all happens in the dining room!

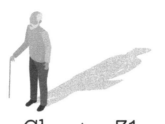

Chapter 31
FUNCTION DESPITE THE DYSFUNCTION

With so many moving parts and different people working together, it's always amazing that things can go so unexpectedly (wrong) yet still work. From a 20,000-foot perspective, all might appear to function smoothly and calmly; however, from the front-line's perspective, it's anything but. Two juxtaposing sides of the same coin? Those in the know might tell you that, paradoxically, despite appearing to be going to "hell in a handbasket," everything manages to come together in the end; indeed, things may seem wacky (because they are) . . . but they work.

Sometimes, the apparent dysfunction may be attributed to a mix of senility and resourcefulness. When residents are tired of waiting for help or wishing to promote their independence (or just bored or have forgotten), ingenious solutions abound—funny to witness but not necessarily as illogical as may appear initially. For example, ladies who comb their hair with a fork or who dry themselves with old newspapers or who correct their vision by wearing two pairs of glasses simultaneously (neither of which belonging to them, by the way) high-light this . . . logic.

Wacky . . . but it works. Nothing but the quotidian vicissitudinous asininities, here.

Same story when an ambulatory resident (unable to articulate anything intelligible and is suffering from advanced dementia) who otherwise requires constant supervision, literally rocks out, mumbling along with the music, with their walker (as if it were a dancing partner) as soon as you put their iPod with earphones on them. This works for about two minutes until their dancing results in irking another resident (also otherwise confused), who exclaims: *"What a looney!"* And they aren't wrong.

But what about daily operations? Surely, everything must be ironed out like a well-oiled machine.

Well, you would think so . . .

Except for when the RN can't get through their shift report without their phone ringing literally ten times in four minutes because staff are missing (i.e., didn't show up and didn't call in) or don't know where they're supposed to work and went to the wrong unit . . . or need supplies (rarely ever anything urgent). And you wonder how things get missed, misinterpreted, or how mistakes are made.

Or when an agency is called upon to provide clinical staff (because nobody else can come in) ... only to find that the staffing shortage is so acute you have agency staff orienting agency staff.

And yet, good care happens—good thing you have good, conscientious, caring staff.

Speaking of mistakes . . . if the iPad-style tablet on the med cart (for the software used to track and record the medication pass) isn't plugged in overnight (or, more likely, that it was plugged in but that the charger is broken), the next morning a part-time staff member (unfamiliar with the unit) must decipher a meds pass essentially blind. This means they now have to overcome the burdensome logistical challenge of walking back and forth from a stationary desktop computer for every single resident—it's the ultimate FUBAR.

And let's not even mention the dead batteries otherwise required for the mechanical lifts; taking even one lift out of action slows down an entire unit at the busiest time of the day. It's no different than living in a high rise and waiting more than twice as long when one of the elevators is down.

Shall we not also forget about supplies. You might assume that supplies would be abundant and frequently distributed, yet from the front-line worker's perspective, it can feel like there's never anything when you need it.

Same with running out of compressed air so portable tanks can't be filled (having then to figure out and call in an after-hours, third-party supplier service); people being able to breathe is important, after all. At this point, the after-hours RN can only snicker and concede that they solved a problem that should never have existed. Job satisfaction, right there.

Having supplies and properly working equipment can be a challenge and recurrent theme:

"Do you need more printer paper?"

"Oh yes, I do . . . actually, no I don't . . . because my computer's still busted."

"Sometimes" it's particularly (needlessly) challenging to work with external third parties. Like when the physician on call "declines" (putting it nicely; surely wouldn't want to inconvenience them) to present when asked to declare a death (typically standard procedure) and, instead, simply faxes the paperwork in. (Incredible how they can assess cause of death from the other side of the city, eh?!) Needless to say, this then places the RN in a bind with the funeral home staff, who insist upon having the original Certificate of Death when picking up the body.

"Sorry, it's getting faxed in . . . so you should get it by noon on Monday" doesn't always cut the mustard. Oh well, times and procedures change (seemingly on the fly) and when not everyone gets the memo, it can result in confusion. Hope you're comfortable in fluid environments.

Or when the snow removal contractors haven't yet arrived, so the RN has to shovel snow and put down salt to prevent people (i.e., staff, friends, and family members) from falling in the parking lot (often, staff aren't allowed to use a back door, as they "can't be trusted" after one person slipped once). Sure, let's make it as difficult as possible for staff to show up to work on time . . . when they're already running short. Genius.

Or when the mobile X-ray provider doesn't quite capture what they're supposed to and have to return. For example, after a resident falls and an X-ray of their hand and wrist is ordered, but nothing is found. Yet, there's lots of swelling and discomfort persists. The staff reorder the X-ray (only this time slightly further up the arm) and find the fracture (meanwhile, two weeks have gone by with no cast or sling). Why didn't they just do the whole arm right away?! It's not like it's a *long* arm.

Or when the team needs to order a medication on the weekend from the "secondary" (i.e., after-hours, weekend-and-holiday only) pharmacy. Just so that the resident can receive what's been ordered, the RN needs to triple-check their understanding versus the RPN's understanding versus the on-call MD's understanding versus what was faxed to pharmacy (because misunderstandings happen with what's being ordered in terms of a half tab instead of dose in milligrams). You may think this describes someone simply doing their job . . . but it's actually someone doing an excellent job, pushing with determination, anticipating errors (i.e., having to think for themselves and others), and, ultimately, triple-checking that the correct outcome actually happens *despite* every possible red herring and misunderstanding—basically, taking ownership and quarterbacking the entire process.

And speaking of quarterbacks, there's nothing quite so demoralizing as those who weren't working offering their unhelpful and unappreciated armchair quarterback criticisms after-the-fact.

Through all this, sometimes people forget that they're all on the same team and working towards the same goal. Burned-out and overly tired staff (from working short every shift) can lose it and become needlessly impatient, snippety, and short-tempered with one another—the very people they rely on most—only then to all cry, hug, and make up.

Providing seamless and well-integrated care takes rather more than it might appear on the surface.

So now you know.

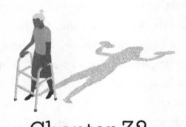

Chapter 32
FINDING THE HUMOUR IN THE SITUATION

When faced with the unexpected—situations that, if they occurred outside of a health-care environment, would be shocking—one can choose to laugh (which may be slightly inappropriate . . . but makes it all the funnier) or cry.

Here are some examples of the types of scenarios—and the means of coping often employed by the staff—that crop up quite matter-of-factly when addressing the challenges of what life looks like as we age and of working in LTC homes.

Ongoing, repetitive jokes have their place—and, unlike everyone and everything else, never get old. Like sliding out someone's name-plate on their office door and turning it upside down. The longer it takes for them to notice and fix it, the funnier it gets.

Often, residents are physically unstable, even when walking with a walker, so inevitably, slips and falls occur (sometimes with grave consequences). In one such (frankly foreseeable) instance, a one-legged (amputee) resident fell. After the post-fall assessment and while picking them up off the floor, the RN remarked, *"We could run a hell of a good three-legged race together."* That turned the resident's frown upside down.

The combination of a resident who is still physically mobile but "pleasantly" confused can lead to interesting events; memory loss and dementia can show themselves irregularly. For example, a resident might not be able to remember that you provided their medication moments ago but be able to play a piano by heart for an hour without stopping or making a mistake. Or they might cry out to a house-keeper, *"You're not with it!"* Offence is truly the best defense. Delicious irony, indeed.

It's not uncommon for ambulatory but confused residents to wander into others' rooms and, in so doing, get into (innocent) mischief. One resident developed quite the reputation for being a thieving pickpocket, albeit not one who was any good at hiding the loot. They would often steal other people's sweaters and glasses, only to wear everything—both sweaters and two pairs of glasses—all at once. For this reason, it's always best practice to have all your belongings (e.g., clothes, glasses, hearing aids, denture cases, etc.) labelled, so everything might all be returned.

Deciding whether a resident has the mental competence and the ability to advocate well and appropriately for themselves (for decisions regarding their own health and finances) isn't always easily discernable or binary. There are absolutely times when it isn't clear just how—or if—someone is *really* capable of making appropriate decisions any more. For example, one resident took to selling some of their possessions online. The staff only got wind of this covert activity when random people started showing up at the lobby with cash, asking for whatever it was they had purchased. Normally, one might be impressed with an older adult's fluency with online communications, marketing, and sales' acumen. However, there were a couple of concerning disconnects. First, the prices being charged were not . . . current. Moreover, often the resident would proclaim that they had been paid "over the

Internet" (i.e., not being paid at all), and consequently, the staff suspected that the resident was being taken advantage of financially. Second, this particular person's judgement was *really* called into question when, after returning from an outing, it was revealed that they'd left in what can only be described as a leotard, through which everyone could see their claggy brief (remember that 'brief' is a euphemism for adult diaper?). A Social Worker referral was made after that one.

How would the following make you feel?

Long-term care homes have notoriously high staff turnover (altogether its own topic and happens for a variety of reasons). During the annual staff recognition event, a veteran employee was invited to attend in order to be recognized for their tenth anniversary with the organization. Sounds wonderful . . . except for the fact that the employee's name had been misspelled on the invite, making them feel especially *devalued* (at which point, the gesture did more harm than good). Careless and preventable.

Laugh or cry, indeed. They'd have been better off doing nothing. Sad but true.

Due to staffing constraints, either as a result of outbreaks or having to put in longer hours than originally scheduled (i.e., you're booked for eight hours but end up staying sixteen because of sick calls), it's not uncommon for staff to order in food and/or coffee. Uber Eats is often a saviour, except for when they don't follow delivery instructions and indicate that the drop off has occurred, only not where you had asked. Then it becomes a game of hide-and-seek to determine at which door (of the twenty or so around the building) everything was left. In the middle of winter, that piping hot lifeline of coffee will soon be spoiled (at which point, one wishes there would have been the option to tip the delivery person *after* one's order had been received instead of when, giddy and hopeful with anticipation, you placed it).

Don't screw with the staff's coffee. Not if you want them to work a double. On no notice. Leaving only eight hours before they're back in again (. . . and again, probably for another double).

Understandably, most residents don't travel "well." As such, a mobile X-ray service is often called upon to visit the home when such assessment is necessary. One particularly remarkable visit was especially comedic to the staff. Mobile X-ray came in and performed an abdominal X-ray and remarked that the patient, "... *hadn't shit in days and they didn't move much.*" This would have been concerning had that resident not been dead. In fact, the X-ray technician had mistakenly entered the wrong room and proceeded to X-ray a body that was waiting for the funeral home staff to pick up. They had to return to repeat the procedure . . . on the correct resident.

Unbelievable, yet perfectly true.

Sometimes, residents act in ways that make you wonder if they've had to repress an aspect of their personality or character throughout their lives. Now that they suffer from dementia and conscientious effort no longer stands in the way, they can act in a disinhibited manner. An example of this was when a perfectly polite, quiet, and calm gentleman somehow climbed onto the desk at the nursing station, took off his pants . . . and then jiggled about.

Other than the obvious fall risk, it was tough to be upset about that one—it was as unexpected as it was humorous to witness.

As I've stated before, most long-term care homes are privately owned. As such, there is undeniably a profit-motive in the endeavour (however conflictive this may strike some; again, another topic altogether). Accordingly, one might imagine that as many items are purchased in the most generic and cost-effective form as possible. This includes toilet paper (thinnest two-ply known to man; so thin you could read a newspaper through it). However, one staff did find a crumb of comfort when they observed that the roll holder in the staff washroom had been placed directly above the heater—soothing warmth as you wipe your ass. Definitely worth considering when designing your own home!

One sly example that isn't exactly in the rule book: One resident took full advantage of the small indoor communal garden and seeded a marijuana plant. How did you do that, bud? We never did find out who planted it or how they smuggled in the seeds.

I guess you're never too old to grow your own weed.

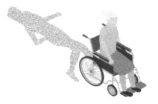

Chapter 33
THE GAMES PEOPLE PLAY

(AND THE UNINTENDED CONSEQUENCES THAT FOLLOW)

As with any larger organization where many people are employed and (are forced to) work together, politics and games will abound. No matter how "healthy" the culture, there will always be a counter-current jockeying for favour and preferred outcomes.

Gaming the system is rife, and for every action, there will be a reaction; however, the reaction isn't always proportional nor is it predictable, even in stodgy long-term care.

For example, hoarding supplies and the mentality of scarcity is often the unintended—and unfortunate—result of a managerial approach to controlling access to the very materials required to provide care. While coming from a reasonable position of wanting to reduce waste, contain costs, and run efficiently (i.e., to save money), the resulting restricted access, however real or perceived, has the opposite effect: front-line staff take more than what's required when they have chance because they don't know if or when they'll be able to get more. This then results in stocks appearing lower than they are, forcing more frequent reordering of supplies (wasting the very money that was trying to be saved), and, despite the abundance, causes delays in finding the necessary materials because they've been hidden. Here, the "solution" has made things objectively worse and more wasteful; you find yourself ensnared in a cycle that requires a paradigm shift to correct.

It sounds like utter balderdash because it is.

Another prime example of a truly unfortunate, unintended consequence reared its head when additional hourly premiums were paid to some denominations of staff but not to others. Hogwash. To be clear, the additional hourly premiums were long overdue and were intended to recognize the hard work of, to name one example, the PSW workers. However, since the housekeeping staff (again, to name only one of several roles—who are just as important) were not recognized in equal measure, they started leaving work for the PSWs to pick up. This then left the PSWs with even more work and wishing they'd not been recognized for the after-tax equivalent of less than an additional $2.00/hour. Behaviour trends toward finding the lowest common denominator. Sad.

One particularly calculating nurse, fed up with not being paid as much as they could earn elsewhere, quit their line, got hired by a staffing agency and was promptly assigned to the very line they had quit (because it was still vacant); who doesn't want to get paid (significantly) more to do the same job?!

A personal favourite is having to pay for parking—which is essentially making the staff pay for the privilege of working—a metaphoric, real-life palindrome: they've got you coming and going. Just like "eye," "deified," and "reviver"—it's the same both ways (can you spot the fourth palindrome in this chapter? Who doesn't love a good Easter Egg? *What a fun game!*).

As with any large building, industrial-scale and complex HVAC (heating, ventilation, and air conditioning) systems are in place to service the global needs of the building adequately. However, trying to please everyone with any set temperature is never going to happen, and with over 100 rooms each having their own window (which may or may not be open to varying degrees), controlling the humidity and temperature is often beyond the capacity of the HVAC system in place, never mind the limitations of hallways constructed where there's a shared thermostat for several rooms. At one point, after recognizing these challenges, the maintenance team decided the best solution was to go round and bolt every window shut. (Seriously?! Was that really the *best* solution? Where are we, Alcatraz?) The resulting sentiment of being locked in the slammer (as evidenced by punch code and deadbolt locked doors, units, and elevators), especially when in isolation during an outbreak, only attributed to the residents' feelings of depression and paranoia. Naturally, this then led to an increase in pharmacological intervention via frequent prescription of medication or augmented titration of dosing (likely not otherwise necessary).

And now for a taboo example (but fuck it): Not all families are innocent either. During times when a unit—or the entire home—is in an outbreak situation (and as a measure to curb the spread and duration of the outbreak), visitation becomes restricted. In these circumstances, only residents deemed to be palliative are allowed visitors—makes sense, right? Seems reasonable. Except that you might be surprised to hear that there's then an observable increase in families who suddenly call in and change their older parent's status to palliative (regardless of their actual condition) as a work-around in order to continue visiting.

Talk about gaming the system.

Same with staff who, when called to be "offered" overtime, hold the staffing clerk hostage by agreeing to come in for an additional shift but only after a myriad of conditions are met (#sorrynotsorry). For example, they will only come in for a certain unit, to work only with certain people, and even then, for fewer hours than requested . . . and only if their next scheduled shift is given away to someone else. So, a call made to solve a problem has only created more problems, and this was undertaken in good faith to ensure the building was staffed appropriately (after someone else called in "sick").

Or, rather bizarrely, the opposite can unfold: a sick call is received but with a helpful suggestion offered that *"so-and-so might be available to pick up"* the now vacant shift. Naturally, this person is contacted but can only accept a part of the total vacant shift . . . but is then quick to point that yet another person *"might just be available"* for the other half. And they are. But only at overtime. Of course.

Now, isn't all that just extraordinary?! Is it mere coincidence that one person got the day off with pay while two of their peers each happened to pick up partial shifts at overtime?

Doesn't take a genius to figure out that racket. Spreads the wealth, at least.

Ever-increasing entropy, as applied to (thermo)dynamic efforts to problem solving in long-term care, in action. Blows the budget mighty quickly, too. I contend that in the end, it would cost less to hire someone full time instead of paying all this overtime on such a consistent basis.

Nursing is just as much about solving tangential problems that shouldn't exist (while navigating through the quagmire of internal politics) as it is about providing care and making sure what needs to happen gets done. It's an art and a science. While Newton might have been able to prove that every action has an equal and opposite reaction, he might not have gone far enough, as the reactions tend to outweigh the initial inputs and do so by veering off into surprising directions. The entropy of a system never decreases, after all.

Unintended consequence: You just got a brief review of the second law of thermodynamics and Newton's third law of motion. Bet you didn't expect a game full of physics lessons and palindromes when you started reading this chapter, eh?

Gotcha.

Acide malo me, sed non desola me, medica.

128

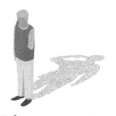

Chapter 34
WASTE NOT, WANT NOT

It's an interesting observation that, as lofty as it might be to declare oneself an environmentalist (which appears to be the trendy thing, these days), such do-gooders often have a difficult time reconciling their views (or conveniently turn a blind eye) with the sheer amount of waste produced in any health-care facility. I suppose it's far easier to criticize large faceless corporations or industries. For example, the volume of single-use, disposable items used in long-term care is simply staggering.

I doubt much, if any, of this waste is biodegradable, and there most definitely isn't a second-hand market for any items, furniture, or equipment. Pure garbage. Plenty of opportunity to engineer improvements and innovations on this front.

In addition to all the gloves, gowns, and single-use PPE attire, it's natural to understand that anything medical-waste related (i.e., soiled briefs, wound products, containers, etc.) is just that—waste.

What you might not expect is the amount of wasted medication and even food.

Much has been written about how over-prescription and the improper destruction/disposal of medication are resulting in growing rates of antibiotic resistance and even the detection of pathogens and medication in municipal wastewater (and, as a rather worrying consequence, in local freshwater, flora and fauna). Scary. But rules need to change before the situation improves. For example, clinical staff are often required to destroy otherwise perfectly consumable medication (i.e., unused, unopened, and well within best before expiry date) simply because it was labelled for a particular resident who no longer needs them (because either their clinical needs have evolved, they are no longer in the home, or they might have passed away)—offensive as an environmentalist . . . and as a taxpayer.

Equally offensive is the cost falling to the taxpayer when staff have to submit weekly, biweekly, and triweekly (pick your arbitrary frequency, really) swab/lab tests for respiratory illnesses— regardless of when their next shift might be. Does it really make any sense to test someone six times when they work only every other week?! Well, them's the rules.

Cost be damned.

Speaking of costs and waste, another medication-related example might include when the pharmacy, for whatever reason, does not send the complete number of pills to complete a prescription (by only one or two doses), the course of medication is made up by pulling from a "stat box." This "stat box" can only be described as a glorified fishing tackle box but instead of spinners and Hula Poppers it's replete with all the most commonly prescribed medications, in the most common doses, required within the home. It's a lifesaver to have for those times when you need to start something and it's the weekend, or a stat holiday, or the middle of the night . . . or all three. Point is, it's there for urgent need, and once you've pulled from it, there's no more back-up (it can take days to get replenished). Having to pull a packet of meds from this last-measure resource to then only use one or two pills is doubly wasteful. Don't forget, LTC homes don't have 24/7 pharmacies or doctors on site.

We are fortunate to live in a time and place where food is in abundance. It's no small feat that 150 to 200 residents can be fed from a single main kitchen, by a small team, as regular as clockwork, 365 days a year. However, the flip side is that there is *always* a considerable amount of excess food that's thrown out after each meal. Needless waste. Moreover, staff get into trouble if they have any. Wouldn't it promote a more familial and natural dining environment if the staff sat with residents at mealtimes and ate alongside them (instead of just feeding them)? Wouldn't that be more humanizing rather than enforcing the hegemonic status quo of the us-versus-them, staff-versus-resident approach?!

And why doesn't the city have a volunteer program to distribute any/all excess meals (with all the cursory legal disclaimers, warnings, etc.) to the homeless or other shelters?!

Waste not, want not—a wise old saying that's more relevant than ever. Sometimes old people still know what they're talking about.

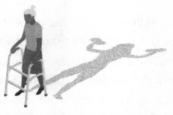

Chapter 35
CODE YELLOW!

In health care, there are a variety of codes, designated by colour, that each signify a specific important event. They are termed this way, so they might be announced (over a building-wide PA system) in such a way as to alert the necessary staff of the particular type of emergency, thereby driving an immediate, measured response without unduly panicking anyone else.

The most commonly known of these colour codes is the infamous "code blue" that signifies a cardiac arrest. However, you might be interested to know that other codes exist for such things as an infant cardiac issue, a violent patient, a critical infrastructure failure, a fire, and even a missing patient (to name but a few). In long-term care, thankfully, true codes (i.e., excluding the mandatory "code red" fire drills) are quite rare.

But not unheard of.

A code yellow signifies a missing person. Given the vulnerable nature of residents housed in long-term care homes, the potential for a critical outcome is high; therefore, these instances are taken very seriously—particularly in winter.

Always an awkward conversation to have with the family: *"I'm sorry to inform you that your mother/father had gone missing . . . and has since been found."*

I recognize the bewilderment that might naturally befall the reader in trying to comprehend how an older adult can go missing from an otherwise supervised and, depending on time of day/unit, locked facility with a controlled entrance. Indeed, one might be forgiven for likening the situation to trying to "catch" a pet turtle after it's wandered less than a foot in the hour it's been out of its cage (*"Come baaaaaack! I can't catch you."*), but old people do have a knack of vanishing like a fart in the wind.

The description given of the missing person when calling a code yellow is also somewhat comedic, and you're laughing when you know you ought not to.

"Code yellow. Code yellow. Code yellow. Old woman. Walks with a cane. Grey hair. Glasses. Has hearing aids and wearing a beige sweater."

Spectacularly unhelpful, really—that only describes about half the population in the building.

Never underestimate the unintended consequences of polite people holding doors open or how convincing normally confused people can be in appearing lucid. Old people can be quite skilled at faking it—and some will try—just like you tried to fake being sober while drunk as a teenager.

The vast majority of the time that a resident is "lost," they've wandered to another unit and settled into someone else's room, chair, bed, or couch. Totally innocent and unharmed—until that room's resident complains that someone is sleeping in their bed, having helped themselves to their sweater.

Sometimes, triggered by whatever memory or train of thought arose from their prior adult life, they'll seek or take up certain habitual actions. For example, residents might go "grocery shopping" in the kitchen, play at their piano recital (and they're still not half bad), or feel the pressure to go to work as a switchboard operator (love seeing a resident answer the call bell phone . . . and hanging up on their peers; always worth a laugh). Those who sneak around, going to see their "lover" by hiding in their closet nude, can take ages to find. After calling a code yellow and initiating a building-wide search, it can still take over an hour to find someone who isn't where they were last seen. When they're crouched in a closed bedroom closet on a different unit and you've got over 150 closets to look through, the enormity of the search becomes more evident.

Life is always more bizarre and unpredictable than any fiction you could write.

Every so often, someone really does escape . . . the building. By the alignment of the holes in the proverbial Swiss cheese, they're able to wander (or roll) out the front doors as a well-meaning family member holds them open just as the receptionist (who unlocked the doors in the first place to let the family in) is attending to someone else and no other staff are around.

Freedom!

As much supervision as there might be within the building, there is actually very little outside of it. Unless a frequent visitor recognizes the particular resident (and knows that they ought not have left and is sufficiently skilled at cajoling them back) or a staff member is returning from their smoke break (or coming in to start their shift), there's often no procedural mechanism in place to run around the building (or up the road) to search.

Some residents will continue forward until the battery on their scooter dies (which then leaves them well and truly stuck; they can't even return) or until they get where they're going. Sometimes, kilometres down the road.

In one memorable instance, thank goodness the police happened to be frequenting the local coffee shop at the time and had the presence of mind to recognize someone who didn't belong. Maybe it was the whiff from the resident's soiled brief that tipped them off?!

10-56: Missing Person!

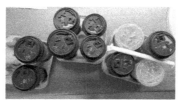

Chapter 36
THE CULTURE OF COFFEE

Coffee—the lifeblood of front-line workers. Bold statement, but true.

It's as essential to the functioning of a health-care organization as hydro or running water. Seriously. Ask any staff who are running late if they'd rather shower or make a coffee before their shift. The addiction is often fairly deep-seeded, with roots going back to their introduction to the stuff during their professional academic programs and training. You graduate with multiple degrees (and alphabet soup behind your name), a mortgage-worth of student loans, and an addiction to a legalized, globally sourced stimulant (ahem . . . we're talking about coffee here, although not necessarily exclusively)—all in the name of *progress*. Such may be the harsh (but rarely discussed) truths of the rituals and rites of passage into a profession.

Welcome to nursing. Not so glamourous, eh?

And this isn't an exaggeration. We're talking about a 24/7/365.25 operation, remember. The staff are working and vigilant every minute of the day; working while too tired results in diminished concentration levels similar to those you have after you've enjoyed a couple of potent potables. If you shouldn't drive while exhausted or foggy of mind, why should you be responsible for calculating IV flow rates, charting accurately on multiple people, or handing out narcotics while your phone/ pager keeps going off?

Yet staff continue to be asked to work overtime (twelve hours? sixteen hours a day?): *"Can you come in early?" "Can you stay late?" "Can you come in on your day off?" "Can you change your day into a night?" "Want to cancel your vacation?"* Seriously. Happens all the time.

Hence the importance of a readily available source of caffeine.

But it often takes on a much richer, fuller meaning. *"What are you gettin'?" "Who's gonna go?"* and *"When are they goin'?"* are all familiar and anticipated questions that percolate with respect to the ritualistic coffee run between members of tightly-knit groups. Some people's ability to remember everyone's individual orders is uncanny (and those who have *perfect* recall are rarely those with the most formal education or degree of responsibility; in fact, rather worryingly, it's an inverse relationship—don't mean to roast anyone, but it might suggest who really ought to have more say in running the show).

You have a very delicate balance to make with respect to ensuring everyone is included in the order, or you'll hear about it (don't want to exclude anyone!). Courtesy demands that everyone take their turn to buy a round (no different from buying drinks at a bar), but there's always some cheapskate who gets in on *every* round without ever buying (yet it's always this asshole who is the first to complain about everything and everyone, and heaven forbid if they don't get exactly what they've requested).

Typical.

A consequence of being in an outbreak translates into further restricting staff movement. Often, staff assigned to a unit in lockdown will be expected to limit their movement throughout their shift to the point where they can't leave the unit or building. This then calls for the divine intervention of the modern food delivery app—*deus ex machina*. Take your pick which one you choose; they're all a roll of the dice, really.

They first landed a man on the moon in 1969, but simple orders and delivery instructions are often beyond the scope of advanced software, data mining, AI learning, and GPS tracking. After clear communication (and in broad daylight!), how difficult is it to simply get what you ordered delivered, in one piece, to the correct location, *and* still hot? Quite, apparently.

If you want to see a staff turn into an 11/10 grumpasaurus faster than the Hulk gets angry, watch how their affect is pummeled when they don't get what they've ordered or have to reorder their drinks a second time. Yes, that's the feeling you experience when the delivery person hasn't put your lid on firmly, and you get a soggy bag delivered with only a quarter of your drink left in the cup. Cold. To the wrong door. And, at this point, you decide to go without because you don't have time to reorder (and break is over anyway . . . and you're running short staffed, so, regardless, you wouldn't have time to drink anything—let alone have the opportunity to go pee afterwards).

Their foul mood will likely brew all day. Watch out!

Speaking of grumpasauruses, once the coffee order (including snacks) has arrived, the day is not yet won. You have now to protect your most prized possession from other staff (label your coffee!) or "confused" residents. Some must have the olfactory glands of a bloodhound because they'll wander, shuffle, or roll towards the complex, toasty aroma like sharks who smell blood . . . and they'll help themselves just as energetically when nobody is looking. Smooth operators, those bandits in briefs.

Imagine forgetting your food for the day and being at the mercy of the delivery lifeline . . . only to have it taken by someone. The ensuing hanger (i.e., anger brought on by hunger) can be tantamount to a personality transplant. Watch out!

(It must be said, albeit a first-world problem, that there's nothing quite so disappointing as taking your first sip only to ascertain it wasn't what you ordered—a devastating blend of hostility and despondency—potentiated by the fact that you've still got the thick end of twelve hours to go in your shift . . . and it's the first night in your rotation. In that moment, steaming and frothing at the mouth, you roast those nutty coffee shop workers quietly in your mind but then realize that maybe they're working short, too.)

Why don't enterprising franchisees simply open up small coffee shops in every health-care facility?! Not a bad idea on the face of it.

Long story short, if you want to do something especially thoughtful for those with whom you work or who care for your family member, or even your resident family member, bring in a delicious cup of hot coffee. Just the way they like it.

It'll make them feel normal again, if only for a moment. (To say nothing of it helping to keep them regular; truly, the gift that keeps on giving).

And by the way . . . that one's mine. Don't fuck with my drink.[6]

---

6   A venti Americano with an extra shot and heavy cream, please.

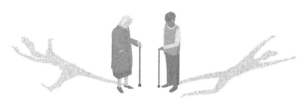

Chapter 37
THE ART OF SLACKING OFF

(FOR THOSE SHIFTS WHERE YOU JUST HAVE TO DRAG YOURSELF IN)

We've all done it at some point. Well, most of us, anyway. Maybe we even felt justified at the time or were simply so worn out that our give-a-damn was busted. Regardless, we're all guilty of slacking off at some point.

But some are clearly more guilty than others. There are some who make a career of priding themselves at the extent and creativity incorporated by their devious means of dodging work; they've literally made a job of avoiding their job. Doesn't that just defeat the purpose?

For your instruction, although likely more for your enjoyment, I suspect, here is a list of tried-and-true methods of doing less than your fair share:

- **Pretend to be busy.** Make it appear as if you're rushing around. Being less friendly than normal (prickly, even) or perhaps looking pissed off will decrease others' interactions with you . . . so nobody will talk with you and, consequently, suspect that you're actually doing very little.

- **Take an inordinate amount of time with any one task (or resident).** Beginner slackers will be tempted to push the boundaries by only several minutes, but the past masters can spin even the simplest of daily tasks into intricate, elaborate routines taking well over half an hour. The guiding ethos here is: "No rush, I'm paid by the hour." Moreover, nothing is ever so wasteful as completing a useless task really, really well.

- **Pretend to be on the phone.** Having props like phones and/or pagers always adds an air of sophistication to the ruse. Moreover, equipment is, of course, bound to break, which can only mean that all the time required to fix it is now your priority (because you're a diligent and "good" employee, after all).

- **Walk around a lot.** Always having somewhere to go is often confused with having something (important!) to do. Why do you think managers circulate constantly (aka "management by walking around" or MBWA)? Advanced slackers know to carry a clipboard (or many papers or even a chart) while exuding an impression of King Kong imperiousness to make it look like official business.

- **Volunteer to be the person who gets supplies . . .** but don't carry everything back all in one go. And forget one or two items, so you have to return a second (or third) time.

- **Close the door to your office and turn the lights out.** Pretend nobody is home. Remember to silence your phone(s) to complete the veil of absence.

- **Take smoke breaks (even when you don't smoke).** Frequently.

- **Take lots of bathroom breaks.** Again, frequently. If you're tired, close your eyes while sitting on the can.

- **Request time away to catch up on all the mandatory, computer-based, yearly training.** You know, that you haven't had chance to do mostly because you've been off work so much.

- **Offer to take out the trash/laundry (basically, anything to get off the floor)** . . . and take your sweet time getting back. Time away from your regular duties and unit will seem like a mini vacation. Even the air down the hallways is sweeter (if less foul-smelling).

- **Ask to meet with your union rep.** Make up a reason.

- **Take a nap on your lunch** . . . and pretend to keep sleeping until they come get you because your break ended an hour ago.

- **Maximize your absenteeism without triggering any disciplinary process.** You can do this by learning your respective union language for permissible number of days absent/sick, etc. Learn what you can call in with (family emergency? Personal day? Babysitter called in sick?) that's a no-questions-asked reason and can't be contested. Advanced slackers will go one strategic step further and learn to identify which days/shifts of the week are the heaviest and aim to be off on those very days. Then, when they next return to work, they make damn sure to divert people's attention by singling something out that deserves to be complained about, thus pretending to be a champion for change. Mastering these will take time . . . so best not to rush it until you know what you're doing (or, *not* doing, as it were). Ask your peers for advice.

- **When putting in vacation requests, do so with a day's break or two in between so that you can call in sick** (again, with family emergency, back ache, etc.). This way you will simply be off for a longer uninterrupted period of time. Ask for any/all vacation days back during which you were sick; don't let your entitlements go to waste!

- **Try to pick a line where you're scheduled every Monday.** This way you don't lose out on most of the stat holidays (i.e., OT paid shifts). Aim to work the least while getting paid the most. Always work smart, not hard.

- **Come to work (and this may seem paradoxical) and then go home "sick" right after your shift starts** . . . because then, at least you tried and made it in. Might as well look like a suffering hero.

WARNING: The one irony of slacking off is that it takes an inordinate amount of mental energy to come up with elaborate boondoggles to hoodwink all those around you continuously (only then to carry on with the charade for the entire duration of your shift—or, to keep track of your own fibs). When the focus is on doing less, the remaining time will only drag out longer.

Oh, and look at the time! Smoke break.

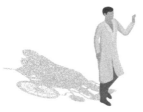

Chapter 38
POWER DYNAMICS
(WARNING: TABOO SUBJECT)

Given the warm, cheerful atmosphere that the (mostly "rec") staff try to foster within the home (it is a *home*, after all), one might be forgiven for thinking that everyone always gets along—as if it's a magical place rife with rainbows and unicorns, albeit with a whiff of poop at times.

Sadly, as in any health-care organization, there's a clear, often unspoken, hierarchy of staff—and that's as ridiculous as it sounds because every person's contributions are unique and uniquely valuable (and especially so in an environment where the goal is quality of life over quantity).

As any resident will tell you, they know who works the hardest (they can easily rhyme off the usual housekeeper and rec staff on the unit and the handful of PSWs and RPNs who provide 95 percent of their daily care). In my experience, if the resident doesn't know a staff's name, they're likely either new . . . or in management.

Sorry.

Nevertheless, there are always unnecessary reminders, as is the culture within health care (however toxic), that PSWs are "beneath" the RPNs, who report to the RNs, who themselves report to the nurse practitioner and physician. Is it during academic preparation that this unwritten—and supremely unhelpful—hierarchy is programmed? (*"Come to XX college/university where you'll get your "prestigious" diploma/degree and develop an entitled attitude of imperiousness."*) Credentialism and the ever-expanding academic requirements (communicated down from on high in the ivory tower) for front-line work ought to be reconciled with its end-usefulness and all the unintended pejorative, ego-based consequences of structural violence that may ensue.

. . . and this is coming from someone who spent nine years in university, collected four degrees, and additional certificates from three different professional governing bodies. To say that wallpaper would have been cheaper is an understatement. In actual fact, given my academic background, continuous professional development, and various roles I've held, I'm often asked by other leaders (with an air of utter bewilderment) why I've always kept one foot on the front line – as if it's now *beneath* me. Why do I need to justify serving as a clinician (or as a leader, for that matter)?! Nothing else I've ever encountered encapsulates so completely how wrong this arrogant view and pervasive ego-based hierarchal paradigm are – as if one couldn't possibly be both an executive leader as well as a front-line worker. To me, I feel quite the opposite; remaining grounded by experiencing first-hand (with regular frequency) how challenging the current clinical work environment can be – in whatever role – can only make for a more sympathetic, understanding, and insightful (not to mention credible) coach and leader.

Hegemony is the term used to describe power imbalances (often the subject of many an academic essay); it sounds as snooty as what it's describing—how appropriate. Often, it's so deep-seeded and imbedded in an organization's culture that it's merely implied; rarely does anyone step back and question the status quo.

To be clear, an effective team needs everyone and needs everyone to work well together—without titles, credentials, and egos getting in the way. Nothing is as destructive or unsettling as a "team" of individuals (rivals) who don't trust one another, much less work well together for the common good of the very residents everyone's there to serve (who, sadly, tend to get forgotten in the morass). The residents sense the disharmony from a mile away; they might be nearly blind, but some things they can still see.

You can feel the tension on the unit when people aren't getting along.

… and should your job ever depend on the approval of others (to the exclusion of considerations relating to competence, acumen, knowledge, experience, skills and judgement)?!

The great irony of the traditional, know-it-all physician is that, in real terms, they're often working only part-time (i.e., when covering on call over a weekend—and for several homes simultaneously) and, thus, can be the team member least familiar with the residents. When they bark orders irrespective of feedback and rely on their station to wield their bidding, long-term damage is caused to the relationships.

As Sun Tzu said in *The Art of War*: *"A good commander is benevolent and unconcerned with fame."* Indeed, if you are about to start a career in health care, please do not get ensconced in the bullshit hierarchy that is so pervasive in the industry.

In reality, it might surprise you to know that it's the sixth "Spidey" sense of the attuned PSWs that is often the most accurate litmus for a resident being slightly off their baseline and in need of attention. In fact, the resulting conversations between them and the RPN usually result in recommending (*telling*) the RNs and/or doctors what needs to be ordered and when.

(Yes, the astute NPs and physicians often ask the RPNs/RNs what they should order given that the front-line staff know the residents so well: what their allergies are, what they've been on in the past, their weights, their relevant lab values, how well they tolerate certain medication, and how likely they are to actually take what's ordered.)

The best RNs/NPs/MDs are grateful for this feedback because they've come to trust just how accurate it is—the speed of trust only benefits the residents at this point.

And that's really why we're all here, isn't it? For the residents.

Chapter 39
GOOD STAFF: HUMAN CAPITAL

When the chips are down and work really needs to get done, the burden of it is almost always borne by the same minority of staff—the true, dedicated workhorses. The Pareto principle rears its head once again; the same small proportion of the total staff do most of the work. Time and time again, they're the lifeblood of any organization; but for their efforts, the house of cards might soon topple.

Human capital is, despite what any company's balance sheet reads, the greatest asset at its disposal (it ought to be listed under the asset column, not seen as a hard cost; the fundamental mandate of any leadership team should be to best leverage and serve the collective capacity to enable the highest return).

Any organization would do well to recognize and make efforts to retain the few (who rank so highly in agreeableness) who are leaned upon disproportionately frequently to carry the day, especially when things are going sideways . . . to hell in a handbasket. After all, the adage: 'If you want something done, ask someone busy to do it' is founded upon this very observation.

Failure to retain these few results in a variety of negative organizational consequences: higher absenteeism, poorer care outcomes, increased financial staffing costs (i.e., having to pay overtime to try to fill vacant shifts; paying to recruit and train new staff), poorer staff morale, and so on.

This is why it's all the more frustrating when "good staff" leave, their additional efforts all but having been ignored and all the while being asked to do more and more (with very little flexibility or other consideration given in return). Maybe it was the fact that a manager called them by the wrong name that finally broke the camel's back.

To be clear, we're talking about the type of exceptional employees who take their needs into consideration last: they will work extra (at short notice), come in earlier and stay later, so their peers don't run short and the residents don't suffer as a consequence. They pull more than their fair share of the weight of responsibilities . . . and do so while in a good mood. To do anything otherwise would result in them feeling guilty (just ask them how badly they feel when they call in sick— crippled on their back—once a year). They're as reliable as a wood-burning stove.

Their values are their value. Caring, patience, understanding, responsibility, integrity, passion, honesty, dedication—the list goes on. Indeed, the trust placed in any institution that quality care will be provided is underpinned and upheld by the faith placed in those working (through the commoditization and permanence of their inherent values). In fact, it might be said that some people may trust particular individuals working more than the organization as a whole.

Interestingly, more than one veteran "good" staff member have shared their common observation that, rather paradoxically, it's typically the older workers who stay and pick up the OT: *"Young people don't want to work but want money."* How do you motivate in such circumstances?!

Good staff typically demonstrate these qualities and characteristics:

- **They train new staff with patience and kindness, invested in their success.** In so doing, they are custodians for the welfare and solidarity of their team now and in the future.

- **They don't prioritize taking their break over the needs of their peers and residents**. They exhibit selflessness and a sense of shared responsibility.

- **They are generous**. They contribute more than their fair share in time, words, and deeds.

- **They have excellent attendance**—perfect attendance in some years and often in consecutive years.

- **They will work with anyone (i.e., don't play favourites) on any unit and on any shift.** This puts their peers to shame when the norm is to cherry-pick the easiest units and times of day.

- **They are conscientious and forgiving**—even of resident behaviours that ought not otherwise to be tolerated (i.e., physical, verbal, or even sexual abuse). In this respect, it is as if they can demonstrate seemingly unlimited patience and understanding.

- **Nobody is harder on them than they are on themselves.** Often, they will call in after the end of their day, on their drive home, to let their peers know what they might have forgotten to do or to pass along at report. They want nothing but the best for their team and the residents over whom they preside. Moreover, they will be the first to feel the discomfort of moral distress when the circumstances prevent them from being able to provide the best care they can. They take ownership.

- **They're humble.** For example, after a particularly busy shift, one staff admitted jokingly that they had done so many good deeds in caring for others that day (more than normal, even), they didn't even recognize themselves any more: *"Please don't tell anyone. It'd ruin my reputation!"* Moreover, they do not let ego stop them from admitting they were wrong or made a mistake, or that they were correct when in a discussion with a colleague.

- **Interestingly, they have discovered healthy dissociative techniques to help them cope and rejuvenate while away from work.** These added insights enable them to work on a higher level, sustainably, with mindfulness. They aren't different—they're still normal people. They've simply applied themselves, through grit, determination, and work ethic, to find solutions that enable them to cope with all of life's challenges. The workhorse doesn't tire; in fact, when you need something done, best ask someone busy to do it.

- **They do not engage in the corrosive negativity of bitching or backstabbing**—which, if left unchecked, proliferates in toxic work environments.

- **They are open to change and learning new ways to do things better**. They continue to be inquisitive and commit to continuous skill development.

Very few meaningful efforts are ever made to retain good staff (just ask them when the last time someone—even their manager—thanked them for coming in). In contrast, organizations typically fall into the short-sighted, knee-jerk cycle of having to hire new people in perpetuity, rather than focusing on fostering a magnetic culture where their staff recruits for them. What a pity because everyone would stand to win. In the interests of impartiality and fairness, unionization tends to do very little to recognize or reward their highest performing members, so they, too, have a part to play in creating a healthier workplace.

After all, you'd think the membership would rather the work environment be constant instead of in a state of persistent flux, with people leaving for greener pastures (typically, when they've been overlooked for promotion . . . more than once).

As the good staff don't tend to engage in (negative) politics (because they're too busy doing the work), they are more easily overlooked. Don't make that mistake—the squeaky wheels shouldn't get the grease. Still waters run deep.

To identify who your key players are—the informal leaders—all you have to do is to ask everyone who the most trustworthy, competent, and dedicated people are.

Chances are they'll point to the same few. Every time.

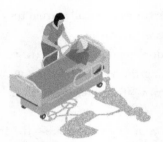

Chapter 40
SEND 'EM

. . . to hospital.

There's only so much (or, more accurately, so little) emergency-type curative care that can be provided in the home. With advancing age, chronic conditions tend to culminate and come to a head: hearts give out, people have strokes, their breathing becomes increasingly laboured, they fall and suffer broken bones—you get the idea. The harsh reality is that most of us do tend to go out with an undignified whimper.

Provided a resident has not been deemed palliative (i.e., end-stage life with comfort measures only), chances are that families will want their loved ones sent to and treated in hospital, rather than remaining in the home to provide comfort measures.

In these circumstances, the ambulance is called forthwith, and while waiting, all the necessary documentation is found, copied, and printed to pass along. The resident in question is accompanied and readied for a transfer (usually from the bed to the paramedics' electronic gurney) and whisked away.

At least, that's what's *supposed* to happen. Often, matters aren't quite so clear or run so smoothly.

First, it isn't always clear what a family's care preferences are. Would they rather their parent be sent to the hospital or stay in the home? Which means the staff have the "to send or not to send" debate. Second, the documentation that's on hand (at least, what can be found) might be suspiciously older than it ought to be; under normal circumstances, it would have been reviewed, so is it still current or have the directives changed? Third, when calling a family, there can be confusion (discrepancy) between what they're instructing over the phone in the moment versus what they themselves had consented to, as documented in the paper currently in the hand of the very nurse calling. Fourth, even once the ambulance has been called, unforeseen delays can occur (i.e., ambulance breaks down or is rerouted to another call that is deemed more urgent).

When the paramedics arrive (*and they do tend to be good-looking, right up there with the fire crews*), the challenges continue. It's always a mess trying to shoehorn their tricked-out, electric gurney (which costs more than a car) into the overly-stuffed bedrooms of residents (the back-and-forth and rearranging of the room is truly a comedy of errors to behold . . . or witness with an air of disquiet if you're the resident roommate in the shared room). And even then, some residents are resistive and would rather be left alone, which, in a way, is completely understandable.

Tensions continue to rise as the staff—the majority of whom are part-time and unfamiliar with the resident in question—aren't able to provide much more than the most rudimentary details to the paramedics, who are doing their best to get the most complete picture of the resident's baseline condition. Unhelpful but a real-life example of the end result of consistently relying on casual and part-time staff.

Then some families have the nerve to *insist* upon their loved one being taken to the hospital of their preference (regardless of wait times), simply out of convenience. Snowflakes. Talk about first-world problems and a pendulum that's swung too far towards catering to the preference of the individual in the sphere of a publicly funded system.

And so, finally, they're off (sometimes even with a brown bag of food, just in case they have to wait to be seen when they get to the emergency department). For hours. If the resident is conscious and not in too much pain, it can be an unexpected adventure out of the home. How very exciting indeed.

"I shan't bother sending a postcard, though, darling."

Most get a two-way trip, but we all know when it's a one-way ticket, and they won't be coming back. How's that for a dark—and quick—goodbye?!

Interestingly, none of these address the larger existential questions (the ones everyone thinks but dares not ask aloud) of at what age or threshold of reduced level of function should a publicly funded system continue to provide comprehensive, curative-care interventions? Is the best measure of the effectiveness of the system its ability to prolong life . . . at all costs? At *any* cost? At the cost of risking its own financial sustainability? (Should we really be mandated by Ministry guidelines to do wound assessments on residents who are approaching end-of-life?)

For example, why is a publicly funded system consenting to have broken hips operated on in those over ninety? ninety-five? ninety-six? ninety-seven? At that point, ought not the focus of care shift to pain management for the resident's quality of life . . . and the saved resources redeployed where they will leave a greater, longer-lasting legacy elsewhere in the (sustainable) system? How might a tax dollar provide the greatest return as measured by the number of high quality health years gained? Discuss amongst yourselves.

The other misnomer (a misconception of otherwise well-meaning families) is that remaining in hospital longer than absolutely necessary is the best thing for recovery. In fact, quite the opposite is true—stagnating only increases risks for exposure to nosocomial infections (many of which are resistant to antibiotic therapy, by the way), skin break-down (aka bed sores) and DVTs. Further, the lack of exercise (and the loss of strength, coordination, and flexibility to prove it), being deprived of social inclusion/stimulus, and complete lack of interpersonal interaction only diminish the patient's quality of life.

Plus, the food isn't exactly Michelin three-star quality. Or one. But, at this point, shouldn't it be about quality *only*?

Give me all the narcotics, ice cream, and group Bingo I can handle. Devil may care—because chances are I'll be meeting him/her/it/them sooner than later anyway.

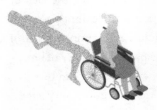

Chapter 41
REPATRIATING RESIDENTS
(FROM HOSPITAL)

The term "repatriation" in health-care speak basically means bringing a patient or resident back to their home facility (be that a local hospital, group home, long-term care home, or retirement home) when they are ready to be discharged from an acute-care hospital.

You don't ever want to stay in hospital any longer than you need to. This may strike some as counterintuitive but consider that hospital—acute—care is not designed or equipped to provide total care for extended periods of time.

Needlessly long hospital stays may correlate with higher risks for infection, blood clots, skin breakdown, and decreased range of motion in those who can't move independently, and social isolation (it's amazing how lonely you can be when there are many people around you, but all of them are too busy to stop long enough to have any sort meaningful interaction).

In order to provide a seamless continuity of care, clear communication needs to happen between the sending and receiving facilities. For example, new medication or dosing needs to be identified, discussed, and processed.

In the example of a resident returning to LTC from hospital, the LTC's physician on call would have to review (and approve/alter) any proposed medication changes before everything is ordered from the pharmacy who deliver to the LTC. Sounds straightforward but is really rather involved in practice; fastidious and pedantic attention to detail are essential.

This process is called "medication reconciliation" (aka *'med rec'*), and it involves comparing what a resident was on before they left for hospital, what they received in hospital, what they are being discharged with, and what they are to be on once they return to the LTC home. Remember, it's not uncommon for residents to be on ten to twenty medications of various doses, frequencies, and routes. The conversation can easily take up to an hour—and that's with everything in a pristinely organized state beforehand.

Because this process is so involved, repatriations really ought to occur during regular business hours to ensure the resident's regular physician is available and the pharmacy is open and able to send everything that will be required. After hours (or on holidays), most can be accomplished but it is sub-optimal. Think: Would you want a physician and nurse who are unfamiliar with the resident processing twenty orders? Would you want a resident to return knowing their medication cannot be delivered until the next day? As the nurse, if you are running short and covering an additional area, how do you remain focused when you are being pulled away? How to choose between competing priorities?

To say that it can be a rigmarole is an understatement. Details get missed. Timelines change. Politics between facilities abound (i.e., sending people back before the agreed date/time without any forewarning), and what ought to happen and what actually happens can be miles apart.

Health care is a 24/7/365.25 service, but not everyone is equally well equipped to operate optimally all the time.

Once a date for repatriation has been agreed to and confirmed and the med rec process is completed, it's always a bit of an unknown as to what state the resident will present upon return.

Have they acquired an infection while in hospital? Will they need to be isolated (kept in their room) for a period of time? If they have not had any assistance getting up and out of bed while in hospital (completely understandable given how busy they are in hospital), will their balance and strength have suffered such that they are now at *greater* risk of falling (ironically, increasing their chances of returning to hospital)? Will they have suffered any new skin breakdown or bedsores? Have they been eating enough? If diabetic, have their blood sugars been well controlled? Have the resident or family since decided to revise the level of care or DNR (do not resuscitate) status? Have any dressings been changed? Have they been bathed or washed?

All very real questions and concerns for the LTC team to examine upon a resident's return from hospital (and particularly so if their stay has been longer than a couple of days). In fact, it's good nursing practice to check a resident's vitals routinely upon return as well as to complete a thorough head-to-toe skin assessment to ensure nothing is missed and everything is addressed.

The odd time, a resident might find it exciting to have a "day trip" in an ambulance to the hospital and back (provided they don't miss Bingo, of course)—but that usually wears thin quickly as they describe waiting on a gurney for extended periods of time to be seen, without much to eat or drink and needing to be changed upon their return.

Often, residents are sent to hospital for assessment after a fall (did they break a hip?). When it is confirmed that nothing is broken, they are sent back without delay, usually within twenty-four hours. In such cases and in times when emergency departments are at (or above) capacity, non-life-threatening issues simply cannot be addressed.

For example, a laceration (i.e., a cut) to the head may not get treated at the hospital if the cut is only superficial in nature. In this case, the resident will likely return never having had their hair washed. In such circumstances, because the cut will have bled and oozed, without a wash, the resident will come back with their hair essentially super-glued to the wound. No amount of warm water, suds, and gentle scrubbing will disentangle everything, and so the care team will cut the person's hair off. Nothing like proudly showing off your wound with a giant bald spot on the top of your noggin.

Oh well, a good soldier never looks behind.

No matter how much anyone might complain about living in LTC (the food, the roommates, the commotion, etc.), after a trip to the hospital, they're excited and happy to return to where everyone knows their name and preferences. It is *their home*, after all.

Home sweet (LTC) home!

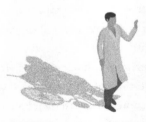

Chapter 42
NO VIPS OR PRIORITY STATUS

It's always interesting to get to know more about the past lives of residents: what they did, where they're from, what they might have experienced. Genuine surprises abound.

After a lifetime of career success, it can be a difficult adjustment for some to recognize the new limitations of their control over their own bodies, lives, and those around them. From life-long stay-at-home parents/spouses to multi-millionaire company founders and CEOs, Mother Nature has other ideas about our artificial constructs of status: ageing is the great equalizer, reducing us all to a more common denominator.

Park your ego at the door on admission. And sense of dignity (you can expect to pick that back up on your way out). No matter who you were or knew before, what family you're from, or how much money you have, everyone gets the same high level of quality medical treatment and nursing (and social) care they need. There are no favourites, VIPs, or special privileges. Regardless of one's past, everyone's got to live together and get along once in LTC.

Beyond the rather comical spats concerning preferred seating in the dining room or in the lobby during a show (who doesn't want front row seats for Elvis?!), most adjust to communal living well. In fact, even the serving order of tables in dining rooms is rotated (so each table will get served first at some point) to ensure fairness. Everyone gets an equal chance to participate in events and programs (and even what they'd like to watch on TV).

Interestingly, families are often the ones who experience the most challenging time adjusting; it's difficult to unlearn privilege and the resulting sense of entitlement. Any time family members "demand" anything, they are often surprised that their wishes are not followed immediately as gospel.

A few not uncommon examples include:

- *"Give him a 'good' dose of narcotics, will ya?"* We always give what's prescribed; no more, no less. No amount of "wink-wink, nod-nodding" will change that. But we'll place a request on the doctors' board to have the dosing assessed.

- *"Only name-brand medication, please."* When families *demand* name-brand medication (versus equivalent pharmaceutical generics), we are obligated to inform them that those will not be covered and that they will have to pay for them. Invariably, the subsequent conversation sounds like: *"Oh?! I didn't know that? Yes, I agree, the generics will work just fine. We'll stick with those."* Thought you might.

- *"Please send her to Hospital X only."* In those moments when a resident needs to be sent to hospital, families may request that their loved one be sent to a specific one simply out of personal preference. Sorry, you don't always get the choice; current capacity, demands, and clinical needs may have to dictate who goes where.

- *"They must receive a four-ounce glass of red wine at 6:30 p.m.", "Turn on their TV and set it to Channel 54", "Raise the head of their bed ever so slightly but not too much!"* and even *"Go fluff their pillows!"*—it's astounding the number of times a family will call the nurse on the floor simply to ask that rituals be observed "straightaway."

We ain't nobody's fluffer.

I'd like to take this moment to speak to the difference between serving and being subservient. Caring is a noble professional umbrella of acts performed in the service of others' well-being – not an indication of being submissive, inferior, or grovelling. This distinction shouldn't be arcane. Let's disentangle this nugget quickly, clearly, and adroitly. We need to debase the ubiquitous misconception that caring is synonymous with obsequiousness. It isn't. Why there's such sticky and stubborn intransigence on this point is beyond me and really rather quite unfortunate. Please be respectful to every person working in a health-care environment, no matter their station.

Still, we forgive these families, as we understand two basic facts. First, their intensions are noble (advocating for their resident); second, as in any health-care setting, the team assumes the responsibility to care just as much for the family as they do their patient or resident.

In the zeitgeist, where we tend to be obsessed with likes, swipes, and the latest electronic gadget, we've come to expect, however unreasonably, instant fixes and entirely customizable, personal services and solutions.

Sorry, that's just not possible—but we'll do our best. Everyone matters, and nobody is more special or important than anyone else. The system prioritizes service based on acuity of need.

Besides, we're all headed towards the same destination. Perhaps you might want to re-examine your priorities in the meantime.

The Rolling Stones said it best: *"You can't always get what you want, but if you try sometime, you find you get what you need."*

As true then as it is now.

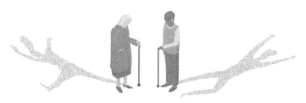

Chapter 43
THE THINGS YOU THINK

(AND AREN'T SUPPOSED TO SAY . . . BUT LET SLIP SOMETIMES, ANYWAY)

Fair warning to those who are easily offended—you may not wish to hear the innermost thoughts of burned-out and exhausted (but otherwise lovely) health-care workers. The following likely isn't for the faint of heart. While these thoughts may seem extreme, understand that hyperbole is often a healthy means of catharsis. Again, it is my opinion that there is a difference in joking about something serious (however distasteful some may find it) and actually thinking that way, agreeing or not understanding the gravity of that same something serious.

Instead of a narrative focused on a particular topic or theme, the following are a collection of one-line zingers and cutting casual observations that ought not to have made it past the stage of inner monologue but slipped past the goalie and into the collective oral narrative.

Staff who work together on the same rotation, grow closer: personal boundaries fade and intimate details are shared no differently than, say, the mundane need to grab groceries on the way home. Therefore, it came as no surprise that when a nurse asked a colleague what they were doing while seated, they simply replied, "*Kegels.*"

Not a bad idea, actually. Move over.

Often, the staff will complain about their significant other or ex(es!) with their colleagues. Misery loves company, after all. As a passerby, hearing only a snippet of the conversation, particular sentences (not otherwise knowing the context) can be . . . alarming. "*I haven't slept with him since we had our kid. I wouldn't fuck him with someone else's vagina*" comes to mind.

Woah! So many Moody Judy's roaming around.

When walking onto a unit during an outbreak (remembering that workers are immersed in the environment for hours at a time), the malodourous miasma is often attributed bluntly: "*What's that stench? All the rotten vag?*" and "*Their shit smells like cat shit.*" Not inaccurate, it must be said (as it permeates your clothes and makes its way through the mask you're wearing). During a particularly burdensome outbreak, a dump truck was placed on the grass outside the front door (a sign of union solidarity?!; regardless, the gesture was lost on the staff), and one remarked, "*What's the dump truck for? All the dead bodies or to cart away all the OT money we'll be making when they expect us to work eighty hours a week?*"

When an amputee resident who had been deemed a palliative yet survived for an unexpectedly lengthy period of time passed, one staff member remarked, "*They finally kicked the bucket . . . with their one leg!*" Funny, even though it shouldn't have been.

And why does it always feel like it's the (formerly) religious ones who end up being so nasty and demanding (and particularly condescending to foreign-born staff)? Is it from a lifetime of pent-up anger and frustration? On that, a staff member commented, "*This resident is a holy pain in the ass. They complain to family [who are overly-attentive and who call in to staff ten plus times a day] about being in pain but then they refuse to take any medication and play possum while staff are in trying to assist."*

Such attention-seeking behaviour is draining and takes away from attending to others' needs. Just like the residents who choose to respond in their native tongue when they understand English perfectly well. Infuriating.

Families who are (deliberately) oblivious or inexcusably naïve never sit well. *"I don't know what's wrong with my mom . . . maybe it's early onset dementia?"* In someone who's over 100?! Those who are surprised when their parents die and have no plans in place (for palliative care, for the body, the funeral, or for their estate) are particularly challenging. I'm sorry, but there's *no* excuse for not being and acting like a mature adult. Don't hide your head in the sand. You need to prepare for eventual realities.

Often, the staff are left wondering how or why certain adults have been given the power of attorney, responsible for making decisions for a resident (either for their health or financial care). Why isn't there a mandatory course to educate (and to set expectations) those responsible for such consequential decision-making?

Another common thread is the disconnect between the perceived, purely arbitrary, nature of funding available for staffing. It can feel like the budget allotted to staffing—the most important component—is tighter than a camel's ass in the sandstorm; so tight, you couldn't slip a credit card between its cheeks. *"We can't approve overtime,"* and then, all of a sudden, they're handing it out like Tic Tacs—all in the face of watching shiny new TVs and computer monitors being installed everywhere. *"Are we a long-term care home or a Best Buy? There seems to be a lot of money for tech, but never any for staffing. It's a good thing that I've had so much practice working short that the residents are used to having to wait longer for help!"*

Speaking of the cost of medical equipment, want to take a guess at the cost of the fancy mechanical stretchers used by paramedics? Well, you could buy a car with the same money—a nice, new one.

You can feel the real sense of helplessness, utter fatigue, and moral distress faced by the staff in instances where they feel guilty about not being able to do everything that's asked of them . . . even though it's logistically impossible. In times like these, the goals of the day become purely fundamental: *"Today's goal: no falls."*

How aspirational.

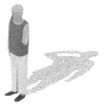

Chapter 44
EERIE AND CREEPY

(AND ABSOLUTELY TRUE)

Do you believe in the supernatural? Being haunted by past events? Ever weirded out by events too strange or ironic to be entirely attributable to coincidence? Well, these tales might make you question things.

Death is no stranger to those who work in long-term care—it is, in fact, expected, after all. It's common for families to find their palliative parent's "death rattle" unsettling. This gurgling sound is the result of saliva or tenacious phlegm collecting at the back of the throat in someone no longer able to swallow; with each (shallow) breath, air passing over the pooling fluid makes a rattling sound (think, Darth Vader breathing meets the "plopping" sound of a boiling primordial volcanic ooze)—eerie for the uninitiated.

As off-putting as it is to witness someone in the process of dying, it's never not shocking to be taken aback when someone has died without warning while you're making your hourly rounds in the middle of the night, especially if their eyes are still open (brings new meaning to the "death stare") . . . and you can't close them (even with a couple of toonies placed over the eyelids). Good old *rigor mortis* strikes again. Always an awkward conversation with the family.

A PSW was once asked to provide a bed bath and to clothe a resident. Rather embarrassingly, the PSW only stopped to question why the resident wasn't responding when they noticed how heavy the resident's legs were to lift when putting on their socks. As it turns out, the resident had died moments before the PSW entered to wash them (that's why the body was still warm and somewhat limber). They'll never forget what that moment's chilling realization felt like – terrifyingly crystallized in their memory.

However off-putting that might be, it's actually somewhat more unsettling to watch residents (the ones still alive) sleep with their eyes open. It's bizarre and unnerving.

But not as disturbing as hearing them, while they are either having a nightmare or are confused, relive a traumatic event from their past. It's trying for staff who mean well but can't "wake" them to the current day to console and assure them that they're safe. Moreover, it's not uncommon to walk into a room and find a resident sitting alone and having an active conversation with someone from their past (or with God).

Auditory hallucinations are a fascinating phenomenon to observe, as are witnessing how momentous events of the last century are regurgitated, offering an unvarnished and sobering window into the past and residents' lived experiences.

Growing up in the Great Depression and living through World War II were galvanizing experiences and their influences never stop revealing themselves. For example, some residents will say they have no money and beg not to be kicked out because their *"... daddy lost his job"* (meanwhile they attempt to pocket bread rolls inconspicuously to save for later, even though they'll spit out their pills). Or, at sudden loud noises (or at hearing certain foreign languages), they are triggered and relive a traumatic event (e.g., being bombed). Learning to identify and mitigate what triggers lie deep within are all part of the total care provided. Often, adult children are not aware (were never told) of these trying times and are at a loss when informed about what's been upsetting their parent.

Nevertheless, do not mistake this type of suffering for weakness; mental toughness abounds in the most surprising of places and where you least expect it. The best example of this occurs when residents schedule their own doctor-assisted death. Can you imagine?! Talk about taking the reins and going out on your own terms. Waking up on "the day" and trundling down to get breakfast (let's hope it's a good one!), only to then return to bed and . . . call it a life. Unbelievably admirable (and to think we wouldn't otherwise credit an eighty-odd pound, ninety-something-year-old for having the balls to go through with it . . .). One staff remarked that they probably died of boredom months prior to pulling the trigger.

Profound, really. Perhaps more emphasis ought to be placed on finding and celebrating the joys in life to give people a reason to want to live (instead defaulting to prescribing anti-depressants).

Odd timing of things and having a sixth sense or an unconscious moment of clairvoyance is eerily common – human behaviour can remain nebulous and complex, even in advanced age. For example, when a resident has an idiopathic urge to make a phone call to family late one afternoon and speaks with them for over two hours (for no known or obvious reason), only then to suffer a fatal stroke that night. It's as if they *knew*.

. . . and it wasn't even a full moon out.

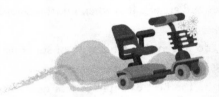

Chapter 45
THE BAR IS OPEN

It's all perspective, really.

When you look from the outside in, people can be forgiven for thinking that any or all health-care facilities are free of alcohol, tobacco, and, increasingly common, weed (or, more accurately, CBD oil; a derivative with medicinal properties)—but you'd be wrong.

However, one shouldn't look at LTC homes as health-care facilities; instead, they ought to be viewed as someone's (many people's) home. It's their actual house. They live there. With all that that entails.

(Of particular note, any time a staff member is having a bad day and expresses anticipation at the prospect of finishing their shift, they can be reminded that the residents don't share the luxury of being able to leave).

Grounded in this more accurate understanding, it then follows that it would be perfectly normal for residents to have access to their potent potable of choice—high quality stuff in some cases, or even their favourite type of barley sandwich.

And it's all stored in the common drinks' cabinet: the nurses' med room.

Naturally, the staff are accustomed to seeing multiple bottles of wine and (sometimes *expensive*) liquor amongst all the medications and dressing supplies (tempting to take a swig on those particularly hairy shifts). However, whenever someone new is around, their astonishment at the assortment is a sobering reminder (pun intended) that people can get used to anything, no matter how rare, unexpected, bizarre, or funny.

The residents' families bring in their favourites and always make sure to label each bottle (along with the quantity/frequency of their normal "dosing"). Failure to label a bottle may or may not result in it being apportioned to someone else. Let's not even mention unlabelled CBD oil (*everyone* in pain or who can't sleep wants a hit of that; that's why its volume is measured like every other controlled substance). Drugs are in demand. No matter how old you are.

However, staff, who, with the best of intentions, wish to provide a home-like atmosphere, must often balance heeding requests for a nightcap with any interactions that alcohol might cause with existing medication regimens. You have to be mindful of potentiating factors and resulting impacts on blood pressures and liver toxicities. Further, inducing sleepiness might be considered a good thing . . . except when that particular resident gets around by driving a scooter.

The last thing you want is an octogenarian hammered at the wheel on full rabbit. One eye half-closed, the other, obviously glassy in appearance. Jaw relaxed with a string of tenacious drool dangling out from the corner of their mouth, extending to their sweater. The aftermath of their driving looks like a snowplow has gone through the hallways: a wake of damaged walls, upturned laundry carts (don't even think about the mess of dirty briefs strewn across the floor . . . and the resulting "tripping" hazard), and injured, skin-torn feet. Good grief.

Never drink and scooter—especially after your nightly dose of narcotics.

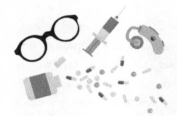

Chapter 46
WHEN OLD PEOPLE CAUSE TROUBLE

When you think about your grandfather or grandmother (or someone else's), it's likely you have a universally generic mental picture of someone quaint, polite, not-quite-with-it, slow moving, and generally well meaning—more or less, anyway. A lovely person with an angelic countenance.

What you likely don't picture is a cantankerous, foul-mouthed, belligerent, and even physically violent person; someone you thought you knew and yet clearly someone you wouldn't recognize. Still, hate the game, not the players.

Unfortunately, the biological cocktail of infection and dementia (or, more clinically concerning and acutely worrying – delirium) can result in a capricious personality transplant and significant cognitive impairment. Resident-to-resident or resident-to-staff physical abuse is not uncommon. In these instances, people shall be separated, police may be called, and the families of victim residents can elect to press charges. In extreme cases, violent residents may be formed under the Mental

Health Act and removed from the home, pending further medical assessment. Indeed, not all old people are angels. Far from it . . .

. . . like the type who were formally clergy, yet treat foreign-born staff openly as second-rate citizens, stopping just shy of being outwardly racist.

. . . or the tetchy woman who admits to yelling out (despite multiple people doting on her every wish) simply because *"I just want to sit here and cause a fuss"*.

. . . or the unbridled, obstreperous, and aggressive ones who will bite residents and staff with all the body fluid exposure follow-up protocol required by Public Health thereafter.

. . . or the residents who are only "mildly confused" but fixate on one resident after another in the pursuit of sexual gratification, or who will grope staff inappropriately at any opportunity . . . and then blame their state of confusion (only to repeat the behaviour). Suggestive or salacious comments are often directed towards staff: *"Where are those bunnies? Can't wait for them to get their tails in here. It's my bath day!"*

In any such case, the staff have a duty to act impartially and provide competent and conscientious care while protecting those most vulnerable and establishing boundaries to protect themselves. Unpleasant, to say the least. Funny how violence in long-term care homes rarely makes the news; staff are just expected to keep calm and carry on—no danger pay or glory to be found here.

Verbal violence by residents towards the staff can seem like a daily fact of life.

"She's a bitch!"

"You can't say that."

"I don't care, she is! And you can't stop me. I'll say whatever I want."

They have a point.

Other residents are med-seeking and *demand* more medication by name (which is a dead giveaway)—*"I want my Dilaudid increased and more Ativan!"*—and then turn on the very staff who are looking out for their best interests when they hold back for fear of overdosing—*"You're a real bitch momma. Fuck off!"*

Charming.

While this extent of a metamorphosis doesn't happen to all residents, let's be perfectly clear, a significant proportion of older adults end up behaving in ways (even if only periodically) that shock their families, incongruent and inconsistent with their lifelong personality or previous career path.

Not all sunshine, rainbows, and unicorns at the local country club.

With the most concerning examples now discussed (good housekeeping), some of the lighter (and admittedly funnier), innocent anecdotes can be highlighted.

People like to keep busy, which is difficult when there's very little to do (and almost nothing *new* to do that hasn't already been done). If anything, it makes the time go by. With so many idle hands and the call bell ringing with regular frequency at the nursing station, it can be very tempting for any resident wandering by to pick up the phone (which doesn't actually allow two-way conversation; rather, it's merely a signal that assistance is requested in a particular room). It's an understandable reaction, given the tone of the ring can get on anyone's nerves. Watching the ensuing interaction is comedic for the staff:

"Hello . . . hello . . . anyone there?! I do hate it when people prank call." (They then hang up vigorously.)

Still others, who have a phone in their respective room, have been known to call 911 and speak to the police concerning everything from their most recent visual or auditory hallucination to the fact that they don't remember being fed (*". . . and the tea is too cold!"*). The RN, who, otherwise, has no idea this was going on, then receives a call from the (frustrated) police that they've been called thirteen times that night . . . by the same resident and is given the not-so-subtle request to supervise this particular person much more closely (not to mention, unplug their phone).

Wandering residents who turn into amateur burglars (never too late for a career change, I suppose) always cause a stir. Why you need to be festooned with a walker, two canes, two sweaters, two pairs of glasses (all worn and carried simultaneously and all not yours) and someone else's stash of ten-year-old magazines is always befuddling. Trying to ensure all articles of clothing and random items are returned to their rightful owner(s) takes time.

Moreover, this is nothing to say of the countless times residents have—very sneakily—eaten staff's food (or taken their coffee). Crumbs all over them, on the floor, and crumpled McDonald's wrappers are a dead giveaway.

Fire alarms are clearly installed just to be pulled. Don't even try counting the number of times a false alarm has happened as a result. This month. Ironically, the casing installed around the fire alarm to prevent a resident from pulling it (which also emits a very loud noise when dislodged) is hardly a deterrent, considering most can't hear the noise they make anyway.

Still, most staff don't "mind" when the fire crews show up. Eye candy is always a welcome distraction and spices things up, if only for a moment.

And speaking of fire alarms, residents who still smoke have been known to light up in their room (instead of going outside) despite clear and consistent direction not to do so (don't ask about contraband lighters… that's a whole other issue). When caught and confronted the invariable excuses abound: *"Wasn't me!"*, *"They must have turned the heaters on – that's what you're smelling."* or *"I was just lighting… some candles."*

Yeah, OK. Nice try, Marlboro Man.

Residents trading their pills or hiding them when they don't feel like taking them is common. Just ask the housekeepers who find meds strewn in the most unlikely of places (interestingly, the residents will, at times, move, or hide more like, the housekeepers' carts because . . .

why not?!). Some residents will pretend to swallow their meds, only to spit them out after the nurse walks away—which is fine until their doses are increased because they aren't having the intended therapeutic effect—only then to "snow" the resident (i.e., given such a high dose as to cause drowsiness) when they finally start taking them.

Invariably, as with any shared space, there can be spats between roommates. For example, in a room with two male residents, one may accuse the other of being gay because *"he's always in my personal space."* (Meanwhile, the shared rooms are barely big enough to fit two beds and with only enough space to get a wheelchair or lift between them.) Delicate refereeing is needed to put to bed any concerns.

Residents may become impatient and ram whomever is in their way as they hurry down the hall (with no clear reason why)—walkers, wheelchairs, and scooters can be weaponized.

Speaking of weaponizing, let's not even go into the "biological warfare" of deliberately strewn feces, where the resident will scoop out their own brief and fling it anywhere or on the unfortunate person next to enter the room.

Might have worked for the Marquis de Sade but most aren't writing a tome with their own feces. Scatolia 101.

And that's why the veteran staff know to bring a spare set of scrubs. Always.

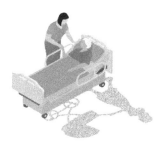

Chapter 47
DISGUSTING STUFF

Know how quickly your place gets dirty and disorganized when you have visitors over? Can't even keep the place tidy as is?

Right! So . . . how would you expect a 50,000 square-foot home with only a handful of people responsible for cleaning to keep on top of everything, all the time? Remember, there are over 150 people who live there and thirty to fifty staff in every day.

Just for the visitors and family (those who aren't immersed in the environment daily and who, therefore, haven't become blind to some otherwise abnormal aspects that wouldn't exist elsewhere), here are some things you may see, smell, and/or hear that you might not expect. Be forewarned.

Starting with the washrooms: You may notice that the linoleum tile is permanently stained (and coming up at the corners). Mostly directly under the urinal and around the toilet. While one's first impression may be of disgust, perhaps one ought to marvel at the caustic properties of urine. Linoleum is known as being reasonably indestructible otherwise, but miss your mark, and over time, it gets bleached (well, jaundiced, actually) and warps.

Oh, and when you're finished in the washrooms, do remember to wash your hands. Every time. Even if you've only completed a Number One. That's pretty much how outbreaks start. The chain of infection only needs one link.

Once you've finished your business (and have washed your hands thoroughly—*get the point?*), you likely stroll down a hallway to your loved one's room. In so doing, you might be taken aback by the malodourous whiff that will singe your nostrils (i.e., it smells like poop and old pee . . . and maybe some body odour, old food, and draining wounds). The stench is particularly concentrated on those hot and humid days (and doubly so when the A/C stops working); it's pervasive and sticks to you. You may want to change your outfit when you get home (just like you used to do in the olden days after getting home from the bars when people could smoke inside). Despite housekeeping's best efforts to wash and clean the floors, they may well continue to be . . . sticky . . . for quite some time. Might be a good idea to have a dedicated pair of shoes to wear when you come visit (and keep them in a garbage bag when not in use).

Some residents, despite being approached by different staff throughout the day, will refuse to bathe. Some for months on end. Is this how everyone smelled in the Middle Ages? And when someone who cannot or refuses to bathe also has a flesh wound that's infected and draining (copious amounts, so much so that it needs to be changed every day), you'll know. There's really very little privacy with such things and no dignity, despite everyone's best efforts. A wound that becomes infected and fails to heal is a scourge, which may result in flesh and deep tissues simply dying off until bone is visible.

At mealtime, it doesn't always get much better. While everyone's done their best to promote a quiet, relaxing, and clean eating atmosphere, the idea of trying to consume food that's been so processed, minced, pureed or thickened beyond recognition (albeit for reasons of safety to prevent choking) isn't exactly appetizing, especially when they've crushed your thirteen pills and mixed 'em in (because that's what you've asked for... because that's how it's easiest for you to take them). *Delicious* — NOT!

Every clinical staff develops a high tolerance for all the unmentionable bodily fluids and by-products they encounter as a result of doing their job. However, most will still have a weakness for one particular fluid and always be on the verge of throwing up when faced with too much of it for too long. Surprisingly, the worst culprit is often thick, tenacious phlegm (and not ripe, smelly shit, as you might imagine). Emptying the suction canister (and scrambling to flush it down the toilet ASAP after opening the lid) is always a rush-job; one look or whiff of the sticky, foul, yellow funk for a moment too long is almost guaranteed to induce a gag reflex. Gotta rinse that sucker, thoroughly.

Another 'good one' that's bound to make stomachs churn is the smell of rotting flesh. In emaciated residents who are unable to reposition themselves (imagine what it is like to be trapped in your own body), pressure ulcers can develop very quickly. In such circumstances, skin and subcutaneous tissue breakdown can be so serious that they result in deep wounds where bone becomes visible (often, these wounds cannot ever fully heal). The smell of infection, resulting drainage, dying and decaying flesh, especially potent during the process of a dressing change, are difficult to forget.

> **HINT:** if you have a loved one in LTC who is no longer able to move themselves, make sure to check in with the care team to ask how often they are being repositioned. Always best to prevent pressure ulcers.

Some visitors and family are surprised to see their loved one's catheter bag . . . with sediment down the tube or urine that isn't yellow—off-putting to all and an ominous *memento mori* to some. To them, that's when the harsh reality finally registers.

Naturally, toileting residents requires a certain dexterity in the staff, or they'll end up wearing it (nothing worse than getting home only to see suspicious stains on your clothes and think to yourself, *"It's probably . . . never mind"*). The acrobatics involved in using a lift to holster a resident—lifting, lowering, and lifting them on or off the toilet and holding them while they're cleaned and have a new brief put on—isn't easy, not in the otherwise cramped washrooms. It's not unlike trying to heave a sofa up a narrow flight of stairs . . . without scratching the paint on the walls. Clearly, no clinical staff was ever even remotely consulted in the design and construction of these facilities; so much could be done to improve ergonomics and safety.

There's always a mixed sense of embarrassment and frustration when a staff member, ten minutes after toileting someone, finds a brown smear on their arm. *"So that's what I've been smelling."* Sometimes, it's a bit more than a smear: you picked up a sticky shard . . . on your own skin.

When residents have a small rectal prolapse (basically where their bowels come out from their butt hole), the registered staff have to do more than merely wipe, they need to reinsert . . . everything . . . with their (gloved) hands. Now, that's love and dedication. And those gloves will now sit in the resident's (bathroom) garbage until housekeeping can change out the bag.

But that's not quite as off-putting, it must be said, as when a resident with a bowel obstruction (can't poop) throws up what's essentially feces (they're so backed up, they're basically clogged). Barfing shit just about takes the cake.

So now that you know a little more, kindly reconsider complaining (especially over trivial things). The staff are doing the best they can.

And please do try to pee without painting the floor all around your feet. Thanks. And wash your hands. Frequently.

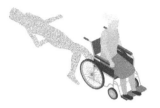

Chapter 48
PRÊT-À-PORTER

The way we dress is a function of our culture and a means of expressing ourselves; it isn't always merely functional. That doesn't change as people enter long-term care. In fact, the *creativity* is often taken a step or two further. After all, a dash of panache and pizzazz go a long way.

For example, it might surprise the reader to learn that there's often very little, if any, correlation between what a resident wears and the weather outside. Sporting a toque and three sweaters on the warmest day in August (while the A/C is on the fritz) because . . . why not?

Families requesting a particular outfit be worn on such-and-such occasion always adds an extra step and takes far more coordination than one might realize at first, especially if there are such requests on consecutive days. Please go easy on the staff when they get the right outfit (clean!) on the wrong day—it isn't the end of the world, truly.

That being said, form certainly follows function with respect to clothing in long-term care. The hallways may be long but should most definitely not be likened to the runways of Milan. That said, as fashions are said to be cyclical, some of the articles of clothing worn are surprisingly trendy, despite the fact that those shirts and trousers may be older than most of the staff.

While some residents can dress themselves (and are always encouraged to be as independent as possible, for as long as possible), most can't, and some don't bother with clothes at all (there's always a closet nudist; keeping clothes on them can be a challenge), which keeps things interesting for some of the more cognitive residents. No complaints. Again, they're old, not dead.

Some items, like compression stockings or foam boots, are therapeutic interventions meant to assist with a clinical condition or to promote in the healing of a wound (or to prevent particularly vulnerable skin from breaking down). Unfortunately, these rarely match the outfit.

Most clothes are old and don't fit properly any more (some residents gain weight upon admission to LTC, as they are actually now being fed regularly, although admittedly not always with the healthiest of food). Some clothes don't fit because they're not their clothes to begin with (it really can be a free-for-all at times, despite the staff's efforts to keep everyone's closets organized).

In the end, there's a spectrum from some people wearing their daily "uniform" (the same outfit every . . . single . . . day) with meticulous attention to detail (well-washed, shaven, and hair neatly combed) to others who mix-and-match whatever they "borrow" from whosever's room they've most recently wandered into (no staff ever judge any cross-dressing). Shabby-chic is always in.

On the other end, others are completely unphased, wandering around in a see-through leotard with a full load in their brown-stained underpants . . . for hours (and refuse to get changed or showered . . . for days).

Those with a sense of humour can find an outlet in dressing up. Once a wheelchair-bound resident decided to wear a black-and-white striped "uniform" as a cathartic response to feeling trapped "in jail" (both trapped in their own body, in a wheelchair . . . and in the home). Funny because it's true.

And real life sad-bad.

Others take a very practical approach. The most frequent example might be an especially groggy resident (who knows, maybe their room-mate kept them up or maybe they've just had their meds adjusted) simply dawns a winter parka over their nightgown—with or without the toque—as they shuffle to the dining room for breakfast. Finding their way despite the two pairs of strong corrective prescription glasses they're wearing, of which neither is actually theirs (funny that the other parties also make it down to the dining room successfully).

In a pinch, form *must* follow function. For a petite, cognitively impaired resident who falls almost daily, sporting a hockey helmet can be a literal lifesaver (anything to avoid a metaphoric 'Game 7 sudden death' scenario). The staff are good-natured and team it with a jersey and a mini stick (placed in the resident's walker basket) to complete the outfit.

Hang on to those old shirts and jeans because, in time, they *will* come back into fashion. Consider this: when you see your grandparents wearing what you think are outdated styles, they're actually *ahead* of the curve. Take notes, and keep their old stuff handy so it's all prêt-à-porter.

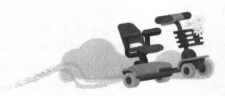

Chapter 49
NOISES

Oh, the things you'll hear.

On first thought, when "old people" come to mind, you might be forgiven for assuming a home would be as quiet as a church mouse.

Not even close. Not even overnight.

Fans of nature programs are always amazed at the sheer variety of sounds emitted from a remote jungle. Why would a health-care facility—that never shuts down or turns off—be any different? Especially one with more beds than a small hospital? To be clear, it's a jungle of people, buzzers, and contraptions.

To the uninitiated, the cacophony they encounter is shocking.

Blaring TVs (most are hard-of-hearing, after all) and residents shouting at each other, not out of anger but from a mix of confusion, deafness, and speaking different languages (or incomprehensible mumbling so common in those with advanced stages of dementia), pierce the air and set the tone when first walking onto any unit.

From the staff side, the global, all-inclusive act of providing total care produces its fair share of bangs and clangs. The thump-thump-thump of the nurse's pill crusher, the strained whine of electronic motors of the mechanical lifts, the oversized metal laundry cart (aka 'the battering ram') running into (and dinging up) every metal door and wall in its path, and the wet squeak of housekeeper's ride-on Zamboni floor scrubber (best job in the house!) all meld into being the home's signature daily soundtrack.

And that's to say nothing of the incessant phone and call bells ringing (each resident has a call bell in their bedroom and washroom; they press it when they would like assistance). The area could be mistaken for a 1950s multi-line operator's room, but replace the haze of cigarette smoke with an invisible malodourous miasma of poop and stale urine. Understandably, staff report on occasion that they experience PTSD-like dreams where all they can hear are the phones ringing without relief. Never mind the weekly (spontaneous) fire alarm "test" whenever Grumpy Gus decides to pull the alarm. For no reason.

Not far off reality. It's an infinite game after all.

And all this while a visiting Salvation Army brass band (that you can hear throughout almost the *entire* home) is trumpeting in the courtyard. Are they even aware of what's going on around them?!

Speaking of trumpeting, noises cannot be discussed without delving into the array of bodily functions that produce audible notes. Moving on from the obvious "Bronx cheers," which everyone lets fly with abandon (staff included, only to blame it on the residents—oldest trick in the book)— the constant choking, throat clearing, gurgling, snorting, sinus clearing, spitting, coughing, sneezing, and snoring is, frankly, astounding.

When was the last time you startled yourself awake after a one-off, rip-roaring snore? All of a sudden, you're just sitting there, disorientated, and bewildered. *"What just happened?!"* It is humorous to witness (always worth a chuckle) and never gets old.

Despite all the aforesaid, genuine efforts are made to provide a calm, home-like atmosphere (oxymoron?!) as is reasonably possible.

For example, the staff are provided with lovely coloured spatulas to clear off resident plates after meals, just so we can hear the clanging of dishes in the dish pit all the more clearly . . .

. . . until Bobby chokes, wheezes, clears his airway, and a piece of freshly dislodged bread flies across the table (complete with an interesting multicoloured contrail of phlegmy milk blended with apple juice—a *vomit comet!*). The muscular effort resulting in a temporary—and distinctly audible—relaxation in his bowels.

When all you can hear is someone, there's really no privacy or dignity. But when everyone lets it all fly all the time, everything drowns out, and there's a comforting anonymity amidst the background noise.

Just tune it all out.

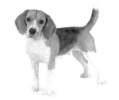

Chapter 50
RALF

This one is for feels.

One of the few highlights that works every time to put a smile on all the residents' faces is when Ralf the beagle comes to visit (the other, strangely, is when *Elvis is in the building*—a regularly scheduled performance organized by the recreation staff). If they could give out medals to service animals in recognition for their contribution to resident morale, Ralf would be up there with the greats (. . . didn't care much for Polly the swearing parakeet, though). He'd have an award for most awards.

His success rate at improving mood puts all pharmaceuticals to shame. It's not even close.

Even in the most "challenging" or "responsive" of residents (who might be resistive to care otherwise), Ralf can cut the ice long enough to get anyone to agree to being changed or bathed or take their medication. He's really a miracle worker; it's surprising that people do not get regularly prescribed time with him, certainly a missed opportunity. The clinical staff sure wish that was an option—it'd make life a lot easier and far more pleasant for many people. His waggly tail (going a mile a minute) and soft coat (especially around the ears) endear him to all (nobody is immune to his charm). Depending on what he's found, his breath isn't overly offensive either. Why don't long-term care homes have pets that just live there? The staff who smoke could easily handle the bathroom breaks.

We *all* know when Ralf is roaming around. The friendly barking, howling (his surprisingly deep yodel . . . that goes on forever), and baying can be heard several units away and a floor up (behind a closed door even). That character, full of personality, will waltz on to every unit, strutting his stuff as if he owns the place. The clink-clink of the tags on his collar and his incessant panting warn of his imminent arrival.

Except if you're hard of hearing. In that case, Mildred will back up without looking and run over his tail with her wheelchair. Ralf's yelp could wake the dead . . . and nearly does, as even those hard-of-hearing jolt in their seat (as they fumble to turn *down* their hearing aids, uncomfortably shifting in their seats to double-check if they've soiled themselves).

Some residents are "considerate" enough to undo his collar—and hijinks quickly ensue. Ralf goes bananas. He doesn't waste a moment with his newly found freedom, jumping up onto beds to give kisses (normally, he's helped up carefully), roaming around on the loose as he knows exactly where he can find scraps of food (there's always a half-eaten sandwich or cookie on bedside tables). Strangely, he always cocks his leg on the same door to relieve himself. You can tell. The hinge is getting rusty. Still, the residents couldn't care less. To them, he brings back every great memory of every great pet they ever had, from times decades before we were born. In short, he gives them their youth back.

It takes a good ten minutes to "circle the wagons" and catch him. That wily old fox. By then, he's already laid his signatory mark—a large "egg"—in the middle of the hallway, which promptly gets smeared with traffic (not the type of "skid marks" you'd expect a wheelchair to make, not even a high performance electric one, but there you go—poor housekeepers!). Funny how the odour of Ralf's "business" blends in so nicely to the rich cornucopia of poop potpourri already wafting through the hallways.

Just one more reason to watch your step and hold your nose.

But you can't really blame Ralf when his tour of duty is several hours long; during which time, he's picking up all sorts of food scraps (and who knows what else) and being held and squeezed more times than you can count—by almost everyone in the building. Ralf takes it all in stride; that's his job, and he knows it. He's got moxie.

Despite his shenanigans, all is forgiven when you see him sit quietly on a bed with a resident as they pet him. Sometimes for just five minutes. Sometimes for hours until they die.

Good old Ralf ain't so bad then . . . and that's how he leaves his biggest mark.

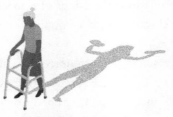

Chapter 51
THE SHIT BANDIT

Bear with me on this. Believe it or not, the following types of events are not uncommon.

Any small nursing-related rooms ought to be closed (and locked) at all times when not in use. We're talking about the types of rooms where med carts, supplies, and resident charts are stored. Seems perfectly reasonable and simple in theory.

The problem is that theory tends to be the first thing that goes out the window once you're on the front line, in the trenches—as anyone who actually works in the field will tell you. Policies, rules, and everyone's best intentions be damned, shit happens. Even unintentional shit.

The complicating factor is that even the smallest of nursing rooms (and, for some reason, they're always literally *the* smallest a room could be; we're talking such a tight space, you have to step out just to change your mind) are often quite busy with multiple staff members, of all denominations, using them for their particular requirements. That constant coming and going can result in a door being left ajar accidentally and, thus, crucially, unlocked.

Enter the confused, constipated, wandering resident—ironically, at the very moment that nobody is around (everyone's likely in the dining room at mealtime or assisting others with bathing and toileting). As with great comedy, timing is everything after all.

And who doesn't want some privacy?

What could be more easily mistaken for a bathroom than a very small room with the light off? More often than not, they'll enter, empty their bowels (just randomly on the floor) of three to five days' worth of excrement . . . and every oral stool softener and motility agent the nurses could give . . . creating what can only be described as an unbelievably large heap of turds.

(On the bright side, residents unable to articulate do tend to present as far less agitated once a source of discomfort has been . . . relieved.)

Having done their business, it's only natural to turn one's attention to the requisite paperwork. (It's interesting how even the most confused or demented resident can act in a seemingly cogent manner with respect to habits and activities of daily living learned over a lifetime. Cues and routines become hard-wired.) At this point, anything left out within reach—from the most carefully worded charting note to the latest doctor's orders . . . to a staff member's fluffy religious prayer scarf—is fair game.

In one particular example, and perhaps not surprisingly, the soft (absorbent) prayer scarf was chosen for cleaning duties. At least the resident was kind enough to hang it back up afterward—before they left and shut the door behind them . . . only to leave the room, which had no ventilation, to bake in the rich, earthy odour.

Consequently, the poor nurse had several surprises awaiting when they walked in. Poor scarf went right into the trash. Poor housekeeper on duty. Poor doctor who had to re-issue orders that were no longer . . . "clear."

Doesn't end there, though.

This resident continued to wander, unaware of the carnage, and ended up with a "second act" in the middle of the hallway, directly on the border between two units. Talk about the type of daylight precision bombing that would make Ira Eaker proud. You couldn't have placed the load more accurately had you used a tape measure (and even if you had a tape measure, you'd likely have been more tempted to check out the length of that turd, as you'd be thinking that that's got to be a record: *"It's like a baby arm, holding a plum!"*)

Again, nothing particularly earth-shattering—nothing that hadn't been witnessed before.

Only issue then was that it became a diplomatic mess apportioning appropriate clean-up duties: each unit was down a staff member compared to their regular complement (again, nothing new there . . .) and the resident who provided the "rosebuds" didn't live in either of the two neighbouring units.

The stand-off resulted in everyone turning a blind eye . . . for hours until the next housekeeper came on duty. Shit rolls downhill. Always has.

At least the resident felt much better—which, ironically, made everyone so much less suspicious of them.

LESSON: Unless you were born in a barn, close the locked door behind you and beware of any potential, cute, and pleasantly confused *Shit Bandits* who may be lurking around. You never know when they'll strike next . . . in the following three to five days.

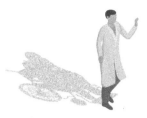

Chapter 52

PHONE CALLS AND "INTERESTING" CONVERSATIONS BETWEEN FRONT-LINE STAFF

(THE THINGS YOU CAN'T UNHEAR)

While it's lovely that the collective conscience of the general public projects angelic-like status to front-line workers (as if even butter wouldn't melt in their mouths), the reality is they often are quite the opposite.

And you thought truckers could swear.

In actual fact, you might be mortified to know that even the most pious nurse can give the grittiest, milk-curdling, profane description— all with a straight face that might otherwise have won them millions playing poker professionally.

It matters not the topic or person being addressed; there are no boundaries or artificial sense of propriety. No subject, body part, or circumstance is taboo, revered, or spared. Dialogue is short because time is limited. Communication needs to be direct and clear, if irreverent.

Below are a reasonably representative sample of the types of matter-of-fact phone conversations held between staff (**WARNING:** not for the faint of heart):

- *"I need to sign in . . . but I've already checked out,"* stated one worker while sighing at the RN at the start of their day. Just about sums it up for everyone—especially when the day's off to a bad start.

- After investigating minor bleeding in a resident's brief one morning (presumed to have been rectal but turned out to be vaginal), the nurse enquired to another:

  "I wonder how she got a skin tear on her vag?"

  "Don't ask. But I'm guessing it was with the electric toothbrush on her bedside table. Batteries are dead—a dead giveaway, considering they were changed two days ago."

- On nightly rounds, you can never be too sure what you might find. It isn't unheard of to walk in to a resident who has passed, unexpectedly, in their sleep. The resulting phone calls between staff are surprisingly monotone:

  "Calling about Bill. He's dead."

  "Expected? Palliative?"

  "Nope."

  "Yeah, I didn't think so. Lucky. Best way to go—but makes the phone call to family 83.7 percent more awkward."

- Clinical staff tend to share an affinity and deep satisfaction to seeing interventions work properly and that they are being well maintained (and cleanly):

"How's Edgar's suprapubic catheter?"

"It's beautiful!" (i.e., It's draining well.) However, the nurse's enthusiasm and intonation might have been more befitting had they been describing a famous painting or a wondrous miracle.

- In moments when a resident has become agitated to the point where an immediate pharmaceutical intervention is required (and every other intervention has been tried), the nurse will call the on-call physician or NP and request a stat (immediate) order for a sedative. More often than not, the urgency of the need (not only for the resident themselves, but also for the safety of those around them) is put into terms like these:

  "I need an order for IM Haldol. A stat order. If you won't order one for the resident, you'll have to order it for me."

- Some conversations are so blunt (described in a manner that might suggest the speaker suffers from a disorder of voice immodulation) that they could easily be mistaken for the staff being totally uncaring (or, more likely, unaware of how richly bizarre the situation they are describing may be to everyone else on the planet):

  "Hey, just an FYI, Edna was incontinent of stool. It's runny. There was shit in her vag. We're still cleaning her out. Oh, and bee-tee-dubs [by the way], her shit is everywhere in the room, too: her hair, hands, under her nails, on her clothes . . . even got some up the wall—and is that some on the ceiling?!"

- Or, when the nurse walks in to find that a resident has fallen, suffered a skin tear, and schubsequently, bled everywhere (the visual impact of which was only enhanced by the fact that the resident in question was on blood thinners):

"On tonight's new episode of CSI Wrinkly Ranch: Pool of blood on Hibiscus Unit, Room 309."

Dark comedy knows no bounds—you have to lean into the uncomfortable to find the humour. It's a coping mechanism. Truly, it is not making fun of the resident, just the incredulity of the situation.

- Universally, all front-line staff know that Murphy's Law of "bad things happen fifteen minutes before shift change" applies to everyone, everywhere:

  "Why does shit always happen right before shift change? I still haven't done my charting. FML."

- Still other interesting remarks broach the painfully obvious:

  "This hallway smells like C. diff. It's rank and uniquely revolting."

- Staffing is always a challenge—on both the recruiting and retention ends of the scale. Even once a candidate has applied, interviewed, and been hired, there's no guarantee that they will actually show up. Seriously. The veteran staff are always the first to point out that nobody should be surprised that people don't return after their first orientation shift:

  "They only needed one shift to find out what it's really like."

And in any 24/7/365.25 care facility where work never ends, you feel like you work short more often than you don't, it seems like you hear about only the things you did 'wrong' and under unrelenting time pressures and Ministry scrutiny, who can blame them?

It certainly isn't for everybody.

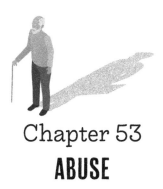

Chapter 53
ABUSE

The harsh reality in any health-care facility is that people may experience abuse of one form or another, and not infrequently either.

And I'm not talking about just the patients or residents. I'm referring to the staff and volunteers, also.

Naturally, and with good reason, much has been documented about the various types of abuse older adults are particularly vulnerable to suffer: physical, sexual, emotional (remember, neglect is a form of abuse, too), and financial (sad stories of family members fighting among themselves over their older parents' assets or blatantly stealing from them). Fortunately, there is much training available for staff and families to learn to recognize any such signs, so all residents can receive all the support they need. Vigilance is mandated, and there are strong Ministry guidelines to this effect. It is everyone's duty to report all suspected cases of abuse, and be in no doubt, staff are committed to providing the best care possible to everyone they serve so tirelessly.

But that's only half the real story.

The less sexy half from a news standpoint (and, for some reason, the one that is rarely discussed and whose importance is somehow diminished) concerns how staff are treated at times. A spectrum exists wherein they may be asked for too much—that thin line between being a conscientious, albeit over-taxed, employee to being treated like "the help" to being verbally and physically assaulted. You wouldn't believe the insults, cuts, bites, bruises, skin tears, and strain injuries (broken bones, too) staff suffer as a result of simply providing care (i.e., just doing their jobs).

Working can feel like an unfair blood sport where it's "Heads: We win. Tails: You lose."

Respect is a two-way street—unless you're a front-line worker. In which case, you can only do wrong, and it feels like you just have to take it.

Is English your second language? You better be ready to suffer twice as much. Totally unfair, but that's the harsh reality; it's okay to be racist if you're over seventy after all.

I'll spare you the exhaustive lexicon of racial epithets and vitriol hurled towards foreign-born staff. Mostly because I feel pity for such ungrateful people, but also because the staff just laugh at them behind their back (their favourite insults tend to correlate from their country of origin—isn't it nice to experience a diversity of insults from around the world?!).

When was the last time you were called a *"fucking cunt,"* a *"douchebag,"* or a *"bloody bitch"*? Or, for the sake of gender equity, labelled a *"faggot"* for being a male nurse in a traditionally female-dominated profession? How about being, told to *"fuck off!"* because you didn't do exactly as you were told. At work. By the same person, day in and day out. As if they are blessed with the divine right to do so.

Residents' families also have been known to take such liberties when they don't get the epicurean 'country club' service they *demand* (in a publicly funded system, remember). The apple doesn't fall far from the tree.

"If assholes could fly, this place would be an airport!"

For sure, some people are just so full of shit, their eyes are brown.

And that's the thing about brandishing an unbridled, hubristic ego and limitless assholishness— you can't back-pedal (and save face) once you've gone down that road. Behaviour like that brands a person and tarnishes their reputation (almost) irreparably. Word of such behaviour goes viral nearly without exception—as if you needed another reason to practise kindness and understanding (ever noticed how some of the most aggrieved have the kindest, understanding, and forgiving hearts?!).

Criticizing staff only serves to make for a tighter, more cohesive group. (FYI: Care teams will naturally ostracize those who don't pull their weight or act inappropriately; caring is something in which they take immense pride and won't let others sully their reputation.)

Another nasty trick is to level false claims of abuse against a staff member. Good thing the cameras that monitor the care provided quickly put to rest all unfair, unsubstantiated and mendacious allegations.

Charming, isn't it? To be made to feel like you're assumed to be guilty until proven innocent or to take an accusatory approach rather than an inquisitive, caring, and educational one where the end goals are to nurture stronger professional relationships and better clinical practices.

In case you can't tell, bullying and intimidation do *not* motivate the staff to give the additional discretionary effort that makes all the difference in a resident's quality of life.

Caring is a hard job, and everyone is doing their best despite every other challenge in their life. Please be patient, understanding, and kind to those serving.

Nobody should have to feel like they're on thin ice or dodging bullets while at work—or perversely made to feel badly for who they are when trying their best.

Aretha said it best when she sang *". . . All I'm askin' is for a little respect."* Even *"just a little bit"* will go a long way. Please and thank you.

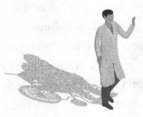

Chapter 54
DON'T BE A LODESTAR

While it's an admirable goal to want to be someone who serves as an inspiration, the reality is that most people with this hyperenthusiastic disposition, upon entering the workforce, end up being a flash in the pan; they have been ill-prepared for the marathon. Having sharp acumen, subject matter expertise, honed and practiced hard and soft skills are all essential, but these traits must be teamed with an ability to be dependably and consistently present, in their fullest capacity, at work, day-in and day-out. No point in being 100 percent only 70 percent of the time. You gotta be able to take all the vicissitudes of life – be knocked down, and get back up. Repeatedly.

So, a quick word on the importance of self-care, then.

Seems a frivolous and self-indulgent topic, I know, and one might be forgiven for perpetuating a stereotype that being entirely unselfish is mutually exclusive to being a "good person" or "good clinical staff" — that placing others' needs above one's own is the only way to be.

False. Erroneous. Nonsense. Codswallop. Flawed logic. Take your pick.

Not only is this stereotypical bravado wrong (it creates a toxic level of expectation that nobody can possibly live up to), but it is dangerous and misguided. And it sure does lead to the fastest path to burnout – because nobody can stay up 24 hours a day or go the extra mile *all* the time. And shouldn't be expected to.

Stop comparing yourself to anyone else. Eschew the meretricious fallacy of other people's extraordinary lives as they present on social media. It's not a competition. Let the ego go. Instead, live in the real world and learn to build and maintain your own resilience. Take a longer-term view of what work–life balance truly means. Consider for a moment that building a reputation for being a responsible professional, with excellent – perfect – attendance will mark you aside; moreover, it will provide you with a clear conscience. Such peace of mind (that you've earned) trumps momentary happiness because it's long-lasting rather than fleeting.

I've yet to see, and this is only my personal opinion and experience, a single academic program—for any denomination of health-care field or pursuit (or in business school for that matter)—which provides an entire course (never mind a pesky Friday afternoon module—*that quick PowerPoint doesn't count*) that teaches and forces students to explore and practise healthy dissociative techniques and rigorous self-care.

Another observation from my academic preparation in a healthcare program (and, later, as a member of faculty): it was incredible that never was there a single class, lesson, module or discussion on financial education. Oversight or by design?! How can you graduate young people into fields where they will make six-figure incomes out the gate without promoting the value of basic financial literacy?! It is my opinion that this is both irresponsible and a considerable disservice.

Without a baseline working knowledge and understanding of (to name but a few) working versus passive income, taxation, savings, depreciation, amortization, compound interest, opportunity cost, diminishing returns and ability to really distinguish between liabilities and assets (hint: it's harder than you might think), all this does is make impressionable young professionals in their new jobs (J.O.B. being an acronym for: 'just over broke') vulnerable to the allures of consumerism and the subsequent pitfalls of maximising serviceable debt-loads (thereby setting them up for the long-term distress of financial bondage). Don't think you can out-earn your financial stupidity; if you are paid per hour, no matter how much, you can easily outspend what you make. After all, there are only 24 hours in a day to work (thereby limiting your earning potential) but no limit on how much you can squander. Don't ever stretch yourself to buy stuff. Ironically, at that point, it owns you as the financial bondage in which you find yourself having to hustle to make payments will embitter you quickly to the very thing you fawned over recently. The earlier in life you can learn this, the better off you'll be.

Typically, personal finance and managing money are taught like a hard science with rules and formulae. Unfortunately, this simplistic approach misses the other half of the equation (pardon the pun) that deals with the psychological aspects of: negotiating impulse control and desire versus delayed gratification and goal-setting, deciphering cost versus worth and the importance of discipline to spend only what's needed in order to save in the face of external pressures to belong and keep up. In other words, learning to balance the needs and wants to today for those in the future. My advice: learn the value of temperance.

Educate yourself and formulate a strategy: *plan the work and work the plan*. Note that there is a significant difference between being rich and being wealthy; central to the former is amassing a particular quantum of funds, whereas the latter focuses on how long you can live without needing to earn more. To be clear, being 'rich' is about a *number* (of dollars) in contrast to 'wealth', which is about *time* (i.e., how much life you have bought yourself without having to work). The moment you give up not having to keep up with the Joneses, you will feel a wave of incredible relief and peace of mind. Take a long term view and start planning your retirement early on. Do yourself a favour: your first day on the job should be the first day you start planning your exit.

I contend that robust self-care is equally important, it must be said, for those families caring for older adults or dependent loved ones. Don't be afraid to admit you need a rest or respite from the burden of care. It's okay to admit that it is a *burden* to care for someone you love. That doesn't make you a bad person. Just an honest one.

It's a long road, and it should be treated as you might, say, a twenty-mile march. Uphill. Against the wind. Pace yourself. Focus on what you can control and nothing else; don't suffer imagined troubles by being sequestered by an all-consuming, exclusionary and myopic focus on work. Build your reason and resilience in equal measure.

This means taking deliberate time before and/or after each working day to be alone, to disconnect and a find broader perspective, to get outside, eat well, exercise, and rest. Indulge in any salubrious activity that may induce a distracting state of flow. Take time to connect with important people in your life, administer your own medication as prescribed, get a massage, and/or follow the customs and traditions of your religion. Heck, even meditate. Whatever it is . . . basically, you do you; be sure to grab a chair and take a moment for yourself before the music stops. And while doing so, make sure you get adequate amounts of quality, undisturbed sleep, and find reasons to be grateful. Overachievers take heed: you need to find and develop the resilience to relax. I recognize this does not come naturally and may cause feelings of guilt for not maximizing your productivity in the moment but if you don't change, it'll cost you in other ways; if you don't invest time in your own health or relationships (as you are in your professional pursuits), no body and nobody will be there for you in the end. I've learned this the hard way – please do not make the same (avoidable) mistake.

In my opinion, most adults do not play nearly enough. Physical health benefits aside, the genius of play is that it forces focus, concentration and being present in the moment – all the hallmarks of training oneself to be mindful, how to set intentions, execute (thereby building confidence and resilience) and being self-aware.

In recognizing that you have everything you need to cope, you will build your ability to remain resilient in the face of unrelenting demand (remember, it is an infinite game). Building and recognizing within yourself that you're capable of coping is what you need to do; simply thinking you can evade stressful times or constant demands won't help you. You need to learn how to take it. Be unstoppable.

But it's up to you to find what works—nobody else can tell you. It's an adult responsibility that you lead and direct yourself. That's how you become an effective person. Funny that that's what you need to be told but seldom are. In my opinion, schools, organizations, and peers are all equally to blame for not making this expectation clearer. Moreover, they will test you the most because they'll always ask you to work more. Know your limit and stay within it. Others' limits will be different from yours. Don't judge lest you be judged.

You really have to be selfish and carve out time—protected time— to keep for yourself. The irony is that being fiercely selfish in this manner is the least selfish way to be when others depend on you.

In fact, you may start to notice a sense of admiration from those around you when it becomes obvious that you are coping with multiple stressors far better. Own it. And don't apologize for it because it's a skill you've worked to develop. Like a secret sauce, you've found the recipe that works for you – stick to the frame that best emphasizes your picture. It's a fine balance. It takes effort to stick to a healthy routine whenever it feels like the world is conspiring to make you fat, lazy, and unable. Gain strength from being happy.

But you've also learned to be kind to yourself and when you do take the 'easy way' out . . . to pick up takeout on the way home, eat, shower, and head straight to bed. Listen to your body. Forgive yourself.

Having learned to identify when and how to be kind to yourself, extend this courtesy to those around you; never pass up the opportunity to be kind, compassionate, caring, positive, understanding, and vulnerable (it's OK to ask for help). Choose to see the good in others. It will not go unnoticed.

Try to keep the perspective of balancing the demands of today with the needs and desires of tomorrow. In other words, strike a balance between letting things happen and making things happen. That means it's okay to pick up OT (to pay off that mortgage of student loans or to save up for a down payment) but not so much that you then get sick, snarky, or flake out of your regularly scheduled shifts. Learn to recognize when the juice isn't worth the squeeze. By definition, there's considerable allure to any Faustian bargain; don't be tempted to give up your health, judgement, and compassion in exchange for fleeting, short-term financial reward (strained relationships and burnout will follow quickly).

You're responsible for knowing and recognizing this tipping point; expect to be tested when you're asked to stay longer or come in extra on a nearly daily basis (it's not uncommon to think you could be asked to work twenty-four hours a day).

Thanks, but no thanks. Remember, being independent is the least selfish thing you can be and the hallmark of a successful, mature individual.

Share your strength with others as a gift. And don't get bogged down messing with the morose complainers; misery—and the lowest common denominator—love company. Don't get sucked down into that negative vortex. Instead, pay them no heed. Choose to be well, effective, and responsible. Time is precious, and you've got too much to do.

Let the ego go and learn how valuable others' feedback can be to your own self-development; however, never lose sense of who you are. Be amenable to change while never losing sight of your own identity. Again, it's a fine, uncomfortable balance but one worth leaning into. Remember, never trade who you could be for who you are. Invest in yourself.

So, when you're asked how you're doing, always answer, *"Never better!"* regardless of any fleeting suicidal or homicidal thoughts you may be harbouring out of sheer frustration.

The adage *"Early to bed and early to rise makes a person healthy, wealthy, and wise"* has never been more relevant or apropos.

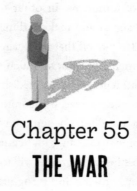

Chapter 55
THE WAR

Tragically, as those who lived through and served in the last world war pass away, so too fades the irreplaceable collective living memory of the period.

With advancing age, old wounds become ever more difficult to ignore. With advanced dementia or susceptibility to confusion, recurrent nightmares of traumatic past events (often buried for decades) rear their ugly heads. For the staff, such occurrences offer a window into a past we were so fortunate to have missed simply by winning the lottery at birth. Often, the adult children of these residents have absolutely no idea (and are dumbfounded to learn) of what their parents describe. Perhaps they just wanted to forget and move on and simply never thought to mention "their" war.

How would you feel, as a student, going in to take an elderly gentleman's pulse for the first time—turning over their hand to palpate their wrist—only to see a faded six-digit number tattoo branded into them in Germanic font (the numbers one and seven give it away)? Talk about bringing something to life that had otherwise existed only in books. A sobering realization that nothing in your life could ever be as profound.

One spry English resident with a particularly resolute determination to walk as independently as possible (despite *"Having lost a step"*) admitted frustratingly that their wounds were getting more painful as they aged. Only after asking several times did they share their story (and even then, only reluctantly: *"One simply did not moan of such things when others had it far worse"*). They had suffered shrapnel wounds (and the shrapnel was still inside them eighty years later) by being bombed out of their home twice—*twice*—during the Blitz (they remembered hiding under the staircase as the bombs fell), only then to have narrowly escaped a buzz bomb attack some years later when London and surrounding area were sustaining up to a hundred *Vergeltungswaffen* attacks a day.

"Those Germans weren't half bloody clever, mind!"

The will to survive at all costs galvanized an indomitable spirit that hadn't faded with age. Guess that's how they persevered until victory— and why the same person wouldn't take the easy way out of getting to the dining room in the morning. Their determination to triumph unbeaten defined them throughout their lives. They simply didn't give in. Keep calm and carry on, indeed. Timely lesson for us all.

Another dreadful story involved a wiry resident who had been imprisoned in Siberia: hard labour, near starvation, and who knows what else. No wonder they preferred being left alone with usually a "stolen" bun from the last meal in their pocket to save for later (a habit seen frequently in those who suffered periods of food scarcity). If you looked in their bedside table, you might find several pieces of scrap food. They were also devotedly religious; maybe that's what had gotten them through. The "thousand-yard stare," described so often as seen in those having suffered tremendously, is a real thing and was observed frequently when walking past their room—their eyes open, fixated. Tragic.

But the inner strength they demonstrated was unconquerable. Their frail ninety-five-pound figure a foil for an iron will that you couldn't find in a professional athlete twice their weight and seventy-five years their junior. Despite suffering from uncomfortable chronic conditions, they didn't "need" any painkillers. Perhaps they'd trained themselves to live with discomfort for so long that they developed a higher pain threshold.

For a brief period, we had two former soldiers who managed to work out that they took part in the same battle in the Second World War—but on opposite sides. Small world. Both were in counterintelligence, each having likely fed the other misinformation (deliberately) for weeks over the radio. They would each tap Morse code on the dinner table with their index fingers and could still recognize the other's style (apparently, as unique as someone's handwriting). Coincidentally, they both had the tidiest made beds you'd ever seen. Always.

Almost eighty years later, they sat at the same dining-room table and thoroughly enjoyed each other's company until one passed. The other made *"damn sure"* to attend the honour guard and, as their late friend's body left the home, saluted in respect on the way out. There has to be a lesson in there somewhere. Politicians, take heed.

At this point, I'd just like to say thanks because no matter how long or unpleasant my shift, it isn't years long, thousands of miles from home with a good chance of dying prematurely and painfully—or worse, scarring me physically and mentally for life.

I'll stop complaining now. You should probably do the same.

And do you *really* need an Advil for that headache?

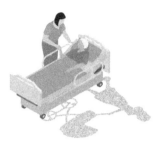

Chapter 56
A GOOD DEATH

A "good death" isn't a contradiction in terms—at least, once you've seen several that are, shall we say, "less than optimal." Instead, best to adopt the philosophical attitude of *Amor fati* –everything that happens is necessary or good; to love one's fate.

When you were young and played the game "If I had three wishes, I'd wish for . . .," chances are that you never even thought to include a good death among the three.

Please take a moment to reconsider. In the adult version, it ought to be right up there. As is, it must be said, not to die alone; I've witnessed first-hand how much calmer, relaxed (i.e. far less frightened), and generally at more peace people are when they are not alone—it's quite something to see how, even when physiological systems are shutting down, the touch of holding a hand or hearing someone speaking softly can make such a profound difference to the dying's affect and presentation.

Palliative care is the term used to describe end-of-life care that is focused on providing comfort measures only. This means that underlying conditions are no longer being treated at all (i.e., all medication and pills are stopped except for those that provide pain relief or assistance with general comfort). Once the decision has been made to initiate a palliative regimen, there's really no going back.

Naturally, the care team will approach and involve the family (and/or the designated power of attorney responsible for care if not a family member) when it has become clear that the resident's condition has, and is continuing to, decline irreparably. In the ideal textbook scenario, all family members are aligned and aware of the wishes of the resident (having been communicated verbally and in written form well ahead of time—and shared with the care team at the resident's time of admission to long-term care).

In short, there is a plan, everyone knows about it and agrees with it, and there is no delay in enacting it at the appropriate time.

Anything less than this causes problems—and completely avoidable suffering for the resident. And that's *not* okay.

Be adults and have all the awkward conversations early. Make the tough decisions and come to terms with all the emotional and unavoidable realities. Communicate clearly and be on the same page (*no infighting!*). Do not delay initiating comfort measures when the staff suggest that "it's time" because you can't stand the thought of losing your parent—that's selfish. They deserve better. While you can expect to grieve (a completely normal and healthy process of unpacking unexpressed love), putting off the inevitable as a delay-tactic or means of coping simply won't work – for you or them.

Often at this stage, people will no longer be able to swallow, eat, or drink without risk of choking, so any medication is given by injection on a routine, around-the-clock basis. Instead of injecting with needles all the time, a port into which liquid medication can be administered is inserted just below the skin. Once in place, there's only a very fine plastic tube that's left under the skin (no metal needle), so it's barely perceptible to the resident. This type of port is often called a butterfly. There will be one for each type of medication being given, and they're usually placed on the upper thigh. Death usually follows within two to three days—sometimes faster, sometimes longer.

When death is imminent, the care team will communicate with the family and invite them to spend as much, or as little, time as they would like in the home, twenty-four hours a day, with their loved one. Most homes will have a guest suite where family can shower and change during this time. Any religious or cultural practices are welcome, as is the family pet (within reason; pot-bellied pigs are pushing it a little).

You never know the moment death will come. One adult daughter was reduced to tears when she misunderstood and thought she'd missed her mother's passing because she was taking a smoke break. Understandably, she was beyond angry at herself, but in the end, she made it back just in time to witness her mother's death—only to start crying all over again.

Surprisingly, most residents are completely at peace and courageous when facing death. Some have a remarkably commendable sense of humour at the prospect (". . . *of no longer having to shit my pants*"). A few remark—and ironically, it's usually in those most aware and in their late nineties—that their lives seem to have passed so "quickly" and that they look forward to being reunited with their late husband or wife (and pet). Gulp.

But can you really be surprised by such stoicism in a generation that saw the invention of the automobile, dawn of flight, the Great Depression, world wars, eradication of diseases, man landing on the moon, and the birth of the Internet?!

Not a bad innings.

One resident went so far as to offer life advice not twelve hours before they passed:

"I've been here for a good time, not a long time. Smoke 'em while you got 'em, kid."

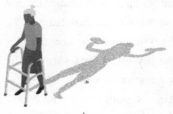

Chapter 57
TOP 10

Don't worry, I'm not going to pilfer from Letterman here (I was always more of a Leno fan, myself . . . but Carson is still #1 in my books).

Looking back, here are a few of the most memorable things said to me to date in my role as a registered nurse—funny, shocking, or profound.

1. When congratulating a resident couple on their seventy-fourth wedding anniversary, I asked what their secret was. *"Just love"* was the answer, provided without any hesitation and while looking into each other's eyes (completely ignoring me).

2. When feeding a resident, she was more interested in something other than eating: *"Come over to my place after, sonny. I'll have nothing on but the radio."* (She was in her late nineties.)

3. *"Do you think it's early onset dementia?"* (The resident in question was in their late nineties; the family was in denial. They didn't have any funeral arrangements made. Don't make this mistake.)

4. Spoken hours before passing: *"You're the only one I trust."* No family or friends ever came. Still don't know how or why I deserved that, but I sat a little longer with them afterwards . . . and they've stayed with me ever since.

5. Being called *"Gargie"* by a resident because they said I looked like a gargoyle. They thought it was absolutely hilarious.

6. *"She's a looney!"* was stated by a resident with dementia about another who was equally confused.

7. *"She blamed me for having bad English!"* was reported to me after two foreign-born staff squabbled over whose proficiency in the language was worse.

8. An excuse from a staff member calling in sick: *"My vagina won't stop bleeding!"* (See Chapter 26 for more details on that one.)

9. *"Fuck you, ALS!"* whimpered a resident during a breathing exercise with someone suffering the advanced-stage of the diagnosis. Talk about a will to fight. Inspiring.

10. *"What's today? Saturday? December? I don't know. What's time anymore, anyway? Unless it's time for breakfast, bingo, or a bath, it doesn't matter, and I don't care."*

BONUS: *"I'm old. I'll say and do whatever I want. You can't stop me!"* Frustrating in the moment and secretly funny for the staff in equal measure. Cantankerous residents tend to grow on you like warts – they're the ones you end up missing most after they pass away.

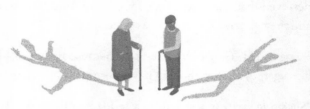

Chapter 58
WHAT'S A GOOD DAY?

I'm often asked what an ideal day on the job looks like. I recognize that every front-line worker will answer this differently, but—at the risk of sounding shallow—I'll take a stab at what it means for me.

Broadly speaking, it's not so much about things being "good" as it is about the absence of the "bad" that makes for an agreeable shift. Jokingly, I've coined my holy trinity for a good day as full staff, no falls, and no deaths (and not having to answer the phone as *"Complaints Department. What's your latest gripe?"*). From a purely pragmatic standpoint, it's amazing what can be accomplished when everyone's actually at work, when residents don't suffer any (significant) injuries, or when you don't need to focus on any one in particular for extended periods of time (i.e., to the exclusion of others).

That said, to this list, I would add:

- no emergencies (i.e., code blue, code yellow, fire alarm/evacuation, etc.)
- no medication errors

- no surprise repatriations (i.e., residents returning from being in hospital)
- no resident or staff injuries
- no incidents of (alleged) abuse
- everyone gets along (staff, families, and residents—in every possible combination and/or permutation)

Each of the aforesaid, in their own right, can and often do, take deliberate and considerable attention to find either the root cause or to ensure that what's supposed to happen actually happens (and that it's communicated clearly to everyone). You have to remember that there's no stoppage of work in the meantime, either; your phone and call bells are still running off the hook.

If I wanted to admit to being especially self-indulgent, I would include the following points to contributing to the "pleasantness" of a work experience:

- managed to eat and drink at some point during my shift
- had the time to get to the washroom when I needed to go
- didn't get any body fluids spilled/splattered on me or my clothes
- didn't get in trouble for something I was supposed to do and didn't (for whatever reason) or for something I wasn't supposed to do and did (again, for whatever reason)
- building wasn't too hot (i.e., the air conditioning was working)
- left work without pulling a muscle, straining my back or suffering any other injury
- left on time
- did not feel guilty or torn by being asked for more than I could possibly accomplish
- was not insulted, yelled at, scratched, cut, hit, or bit

All in all, I do not believe that it takes anything unreasonable to make for a good day. Heck, I didn't even ask to get thanked or recognized for managing to pull off a logistical miracle, as is so often required.

I'm sure most others would set the bar equally low.

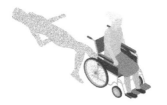

Chapter 59
IDYLLIC FUTURE STATE

Whenever you find yourself in a room full of overly enthusiastic change-management zealots, they speak to "idyllic future states" as this utopia of what life at work could be like. I suppose it's a motivating tactic to drive everyone else to do the work. You need to "create a sense of urgency" to "inspire people to act" . . . or so says the tenet (as if people can't see right through it). Regardless, it's a question that crops up and—at the advice of several people, not least of all my editor and publisher—I thought it important to include with respect to how I'd like to see the state of LTC.

Again, this is nothing but a personal opinion and is presented in no particular order. I am not trying to be a harbinger, pontificating or meaning to be instructional. My purpose here is merely to conceptualize and promote a future state that might be more meaningful to all stakeholders. I've never been someone concerned with people's perceptions over sense and end-user value; to me, optics are politically motivated rather than a preference for action based on an authentic desire to move the needle.

First, a level playing field for the staff should be created. Well begun is half done. This would mean (through whatever means—legislation, if necessary) that regardless of where you work, you could expect the same pay. Unsurprisingly, it's especially difficult to recruit and retain in LTC when you get paid more pretty much everywhere else—for almost any equivalent role—from front-line clinicians to management and executive leadership. Equal pay would mean not only recognizing concurrent experience of staff (so they can climb experience-based pay scales according to their true total of working hours) but also matching hourly shift premiums and rates of OT and stat pay. Small steps in this area would be no small thing.

Second, there would have to be a boom in new construction; you simply can't retrofit older buildings beyond a certain point. Really old buildings ought to be shut down. Better temperature control and ventilation inside buildings are both needed. As is greater capacity and flexibility to provide positive and negative pressure rooms with higher rates of appropriately filtered ventilation (measured in number of air exchanges per hour). Enhanced ability to stop the spread of infections and prevent outbreaks really begin within the confines, layouts, and spacing of the physical environment; the up-front cost of construction would be paid back quickly with better health outcomes (i.e., reducing the rate of communicable illnesses and resulting hospital admissions).

Third, higher quality, healthier food should be provided and less processed, carb-loaded, sugary snacks given. More vegetarian/vegan-based options would be good too. To add, if tangentially, would be additional resources to enable deliberate efforts on maintaining optimal oral health; too many people's teeth are left to rot. This is preventable.

Fourth, there should be a greater focus on environmentalism (and I'm truly not a tree hugger). There's tremendous potential for industry research and development here; the amount of one-time use disposable products is staggering.

Fifth, there should be a renewed emphasis on the importance of exercise and more resources to promote, nudge, and facilitate residents' efforts to keep active for as long as possible: more walking (or rolling), more stretching, more strength-based exercises, and less sitting around. Combine this with a push for more frequent opportunities for residents to spend time outside. The fact that an LTC home may have a courtyard speaks more to the ideas of optics and moral licensing than a commitment to have it put to fullest, regular, and sustained use.

Sixth, to piggy-back off the root of previous point, every home should have at least one person (more would be better; heck, strike up a 'listening committee'), whose job it would be to sit and spend time to listen to each resident. Educating all staff and families on the importance of being patient and creating a safe space for residents to speak would be profound. In particular, those residents who might be especially anxious or who come from distressing backgrounds might stand to benefit most from the opportunity to talk and feel heard without being rushed. The sad truth is that the clinical staff rarely have the time to do this, as much as they would like to do so. Without any agenda or judgement, the wisdom, anecdotes or insights to be gleaned would demonstrate acceptance, love and respect for the lives lived; I'd wager that the clinical staff and families would stand to learn more than they bargained for while care outcomes (particularly for mental health issues) could only benefit from this simple yet powerful intervention. Listening – who knew?!

Seven, wherever possible, create a dedicated space for live-in animals. A dog. A cat. Couple of rabbits. You get the idea. Basically, a safe space – engineered correctly (thinking: proper ventilation, easy access to hand-washing, fall risk reduction and basic infection control measures in place) – where any resident (and family) could visit to their hearts' content. A welcome distraction where fond memories and easy smiles would abound.

Eight, offering education to families or anyone acting as the POA (and even executor to a will) to let them know what to expect—and what is expected of them. For example, what to have organized, how to set realistic expectations, and who to call for what and when. This will familiarize everyone with how the "system" works, so they can engage meaningfully and advocate more effectively, rather than feel left on the sidelines.

Next, the area could do with having less of a litigious flavour. As has been of increasing *de rigueur* of best practices in health care over the past several decades, everyone seems to be more concerned about papering themselves with a proliferation of required documentation to the exclusion of being present to provide good care. All this in the name of CYA (or, to CYA for the organization). Talk about not seeing the forest for the trees. I'm not advocating for not having standards or for not being accountable, but if you spend more time documenting than you do providing care and being available to be hands-on, doesn't that defeat the point? Since when is it more important to sit alone at a computer screen than to help someone face-to-face? Again, the harmful externality of "necessary" documentation results in a dearth of time to promote resident wellness (which, ironically, would result in a vortex of still more documentation) and more frequent poorer health outcomes.

Last, and this is the tough one, have a larger discussion on what end-of-life means and become comfortable with death. This will require education. I would like to see a mental shift in default clinical focus from treatment to quality of life. Why are we giving eighty-year-olds fifteen pills every morning but can't get them meaningful one-on-one time every day with someone to talk to for more than five minutes? Why can't there be recreation staff, exercise staff, and pet therapy for everyone every day?! I know it's not easy, and I'm not advocating that we simply stop treating chronic conditions, but I believe the current point of balance is off; people should receive only what's absolutely necessary to be comfortable. The primary goal ought not be to prolong life but to make it as painless and pleasant as possible. I don't think there are any Ministry standards on resident happiness (and I could be wrong)—but there should be. If your residents don't score at least "7/10 happy" on average, then you're doing something wrong. Or not doing something right. Or not really doing much of anything beyond simply warehousing them.

But that's just my $0.02.

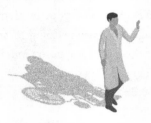

POSTSCRIPT

Thank you for having taken the time to read this collection of topic-based short stories. Maybe you've learned a thing or two. Hopefully, you'll feel you've gained broader insight into the various facets of life and the global experience of long-term care from several unvarnished points of view.

Good writing means telling the truth, and finding out how people work, live, and die is important. We need to stop treating dying and death as taboo subjects. Life goes on right until the end, and it can be, at times, *really* funny. Stay buoyant during the (flat-lining) process and share your strength with others as a gift. Don't be terrified of aging and death—shake off the solemnity and look for the good.

For example, while caring for a palliative resident, I will often advise the family to watch their loved one carefully because anyone who is dying actively is actually forcing us to confront how to live. Conceptualize that how you elect to spend your time as choosing to purchase the moment with your life. To this end, re-examine your habits as they do tend to add up and make you who you are. Moreover, death isn't really a future occurrence—it happens every day because nobody can get time back; each day is unrepeatable. Seneca said (I'm paraphrasing here; I didn't actually hear him say this. . .): "Time that passes belongs to death."

Remember this when you're struggling: live like you are dying because we're all terminal. Force yourself to make the rest of your life, the best of your life.

Perhaps I've made the mistake of assuming that everything that's happened to me is interesting (or so unbelievably crazy, it just had to be told). Regardless, in the end, I hope this book will raise awareness and help others in similar situations.

I wrote as if nobody would read this (statistically speaking, as a first-time author, there is considerable evidence to support this assumption), which made it all the easier to not hold back and to tell it like it really is. Life and work in long-term care is not easy and can be surreally fucked up. However, it can be dignified and peaceful, also. By nature, I'm a congenial pessimist: I'm friendly to everyone but expect the worst—so I won't be offended if this book rubbed you the wrong way.

If you're a student going into any facet of health care, I hope you have developed a greater appreciation for what you're getting yourself into (like, what you're *really* getting yourself into). Perhaps you'll even find this work more informative than some of your assigned readings from curricular textbooks. The dark and "sad-bad" (not so nicey-nicey) side of health care is this: it simply isn't fun, and there's a lot that's not okay—to describe it otherwise would be inauthentic. I strongly advise against pursuing a career in health care for ego-based reasons of presumed glamour, status, or financial reward.

But if you do delve in, my advice is this: learn and practise healthy dissociative techniques to keep yourself from getting rundown and burned out—from Day One. Robust self-care is essential, and professional schools rarely do a good job of nurturing such skills. Now, put this book down, go for a run, shower, eat some veggies, and go to bed early. Work is a marathon, not a sprint. Learn to pace yourself. You're of no use to anyone—your patients or colleagues—and you can't expect to give of yourself to provide good care day in and day out if you're not looking after yourself first. Always.

If you have a parent or loved one in LTC (or about to be admitted), you will have a more fulsome understanding now of the constellation of factors and types of experiences they likely encounter on the daily. Additionally, you've picked up a tip or two on how to be most effectively involved in the life of "your" resident. These stories should provide plenty to talk about when you visit or speak with them next.

If you are a veteran health-care worker, you will have been able to identify with any number of these stories (you know that real life can be, and often is, stranger than any fiction) and find that you are less alone in living the work life you do. In these shared experiences, you will find support. In laughing at your work life, there is therapy.

If you are a family member of a health-care worker, this should have provided you with insight into what they face every day—and why they're so cranky, hungry, frustrated, or exhausted when they get home. Maybe it's because they've had a bad day that they don't want to talk . . . or maybe they do. But at least now you know where they might be coming from (and the kinds of things they can't unsee or unhear).

Last, if you have been in an LTC home for a while, you can both identify and laugh at how crazy the "zoo" may seem at times. But if you're about to be admitted to LTC, there's lots to look forward to, which is so rarely emphasized. With something always going on, there's never a dull moment despite the hours of boredom at *The Wrinkly Ranch*.

ACKNOWLEDGEMENTS

I am grateful to the non-judgmental handful of supportive people who helped get this passion project off the ground and onto the page. Thank you for being so patient and humouring me; I imagine it must have been like indulging a small child who had just learned a simple magic trick— *really* annoying a lot of the time. Thank you for holding me accountable and my feet to the fire to keep producing—that was clutch. And, most of all, for challenging me when what I was writing was utter crap, off-topic, or for reining me in when it was simply unpublishable. Your unwavering tolerance and encouragement are recognized and sincerely appreciated.

I won't name you . . . so you can save face and not go down with the ship. But you know who you are. And you're really important to me.

Thanks again.

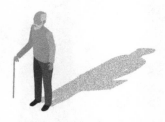

COMMON ABBREVIATIONS & ACRONYMS

ADLs	activities of daily living
ALS	amyotrophic lateral sclerosis (a progressive neurological disease that causes increasing loss of muscle control; often referred to as Lou Gehrig's disease)
BID	twice a day
BM	bowel movement (e.g., taking a crap)
BP	blood pressure
C. diff	Clostridium difficile. Bacterial infection (CDI) in the intestine that produces a toxin and causes potentially dangerous diarrhea and colitis
CBI	continuous bladder irrigation
CHF	congestive heart failure
COPD	chronic obstructive pulmonary disease
CPR	cardio pulmonary resuscitation
CQI	continuous quality improvement
CVA	cerebrovascular accident (e.g., a stroke)
CYA	cover your ass
DM	diabetes mellitus

DNR	do not resuscitate
DVT	deep vein thrombosis (when a blot clot clogs a major vein)
Dx	diagnosis
FH	funeral home
FLI	flu-like illness
FLK	"funny-looking" kid
FML	fuck my life
FUBAR	fucked up beyond all reason
GFY	Go fuck yourself!
gtts	drops (usually for eyes)
HS	at bedtime
HVAC	heating, ventilation, and air conditioning
Hx	history
IDGARA	I don't give a rat's ass
IM	intramuscularly
IV	intravenous
KPIs	key performance indicators
LE	life enrichment (aka *rec staff*)
LTC or LTCH	long-term care home
MBWA	management by walking around (a great tactic to appear visible and busy without doing much of anything of any value)
MD	medical doctor
MI	myocardial infarction (e.g., heart attack)
MMSE	Mini-Mental State Exam
MRSA	methicillin-resistant staphylococcus aureus
np	nasopharyngeal (or, 'NP' for 'NP swab')
NP	nurse practitioner
NPO	nothing by mouth
OB	outbreak
OD	right eye

OG	original gangster (typically in reference of the first person/thing to have done something that has since been accepted as standard or copied)
OS	left eye
OT	occupational therapy and also overtime (typically paid at one and a half times normal hourly rate, but may be up to two to three times)
OTB	on the ball
OU	both eyes
PCR	polymerase chain reaction (a highly accurate genetic test used to confirm if a pathogen is present in a sample; e.g., COVID in an NP swab)
PE	pulmonary embolism (when a blot clot clogs an artery in the lung)
PH	Public Health
PICC	peripherally inserted central catheter
POA	power of attorney
po	by mouth
PPE	personal protective equipment
PRN	as needed (e.g., a medication that can be given in addition to what is regularly scheduled)
pr	per rectum (i.e., up the bum)
PSW	personal support worker
PT	physiotherapy
PTSD	post-traumatic stress disorder
pv	per vagina (i.e., up the vag)
QAM	every morning
QD	every day
QID	four times a day
RBF	resting bitch face (if you see this look on someone, proceed with *extreme* caution)
RH	retirement home

RN	registered nurse
RPN	registered practical nurse
Rx	prescription
sc	subcutaneously (i.e., under the skin)
stat	immediately (from the Latin *statim*); usually in reference to a one-time (additional dose) of medication to be given right away
stats	"stat" or statuary holiday (a day where, when worked, staff are paid at OT rate)
STIs	sexually transmitted infections (previously referred to as STDs)
SW	social worker
TB	tuberculosis
TIA	transient ischemic attack (colloquially known as a mini stroke; it will usually resolve on its own but is to be taken seriously and as a sign that further assessments are warranted)
TID	three times a day
UTI	urinary tract infection
VPDs	vaccine preventable diseases
VRE	vancomycin-resistant enterococci
XR	X-ray[7]

---

7   . . . hope all that isn't TMI.

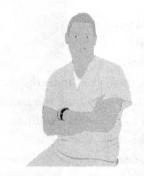

ABOUT THE AUTHOR

Tristan Squire-Smith is a Registered Nurse with a constellation of professional experiences having served in leadership positions, academic lecturing and clinical instruction appointments, and front-line nursing work in medicine, long-term care (LTC), mental health and public health environments. Holding degrees in chemistry, modern languages, nursing and a Master's of Business Administration, and having obtained the Certification Board of Infection Control and Epidemiology's Certification of Infection Control (CIC) and The Canadian College of Health Leaders' Certified Health Executive (CHE) designation, have enabled Tristan to manage teams and lead organizations in both the public and private sectors. He continues to work on the front line in LTC, provides business-related consulting services, has achieved patent-pending status with the United States Patent and Trademark Office with his proprietary infection-preventing water activity and sport related product, and recently earned his real estate license. *The Wrinkly Ranch* is Tristan's first book.

For more information, please visit: www.thewrinklyranch.com

CPSIA information can be obtained
at www.ICGtesting.com
Printed in the USA
LVHW010212150822
725929LV00004B/309